íc

Quiet Killers

Quiet Killers

The Fall and Rise of Deadly Diseases

DR ROBERT BAKER

Foreword by Dr Phil Hammond

SUTTON PUBLISHING

First published in the United Kingdom in 2007 by
Sutton Publishing Limited · Phoenix Mill
Thrupp · Stroud · Gloucestershire · GL5 2BU

British Library Cataloguing in Publication Data
A catalogue record for this book is available from the British Library.

Hardback ISBN 978-0-7509-4108-2
Paperback ISBN 978-0-7509-4109-9

Typeset in Sabon.
Typesetting and origination by
Sutton Publishing Limited.
Printed and bound in England by
J.H. Haynes & Co. Ltd, Sparkford.

Contents

List of Illustrations

Foreword

Do you communicate better than your bacteria? If you grunt behind the newspaper and drip marmalade down your tie, the chances are you don't. As Robert Baker puts it, 'Would it surprise you to learn that bacteria live, often harmoniously, in multiracial communities? That they talk to each other? Hold board meetings to decide on plans of action? Feed each other? Fight each other? Protect each other? Sleep? Share news and information? Pass on tips for fighting antibiotics? They even talk to you, and you talk back to them. Each of us is in a state of continuous conversation with the bacteria that share our lives, determining whether we live in a state of truce or war.'

Dr Baker writes as he speaks, and reading *Quiet Killers* is akin to having an erudite and witty physician delivering a lantern lecture in your front room. But the beauty of the book lies in Baker's enthusiasm for his subject. He has unashamedly cherry-picked the most riveting facets of infectious disease and placed them in historical, social and global contexts. The result is fascinating.

Viruses and bacteria are quiet killers in the sense that they often fly under the radar and only reveal themselves to us when it is too late for our immune system to put up much of a fight. And they quietly bide their time, lulling us into the false sense of security that they have receded, before mounting a devastating comeback. To each other, they are loud and raucous, and they might be to us if only we listened. Alas, we usually ignore them and fail to learn the lessons of history and evolution. Baker illustrates beautifully how many of today's epidemics are predictable.

Infectious diseases have altered the course of history far more than our lame attempts at war. But they are not all bad. Their evolutionary challenge has helped us to evolve. As Baker says, 'We are essentially composed of microbes living in huge communities with the emergent properties of life and consciousness.' Our relationship with our bugs is highly complex. We contain billions of organisms that live harmoniously in one part of our body, but which could easily kill us if they ended up in another.

Quiet Killers is full of fighting talk. Our struggle with them over the centuries has delivered some 'haymaker blows', but as yet no knockout. The struggle is akin to 'an ungloved boxing match between two prize-fighters'. But the lasting impression is to be in awe of the fiendish evolutionary ingenuity that has allowed these organisms to adapt, survive and flourish in the face of all we have thrown at them. Yes, they can kill us, but often because our fickleness, selfishness and short memories have allowed them to. We don't just need to read this book; we need to digest it before the next quiet killer digests us.

Dr Phil Hammond

Acknowledgements

I would like to acknowledge the skilled editorial assistance of Commissioning Editor at Sutton Jaqueline Mitchell. Thank you also to my agent, Charlotte Howard of Fox and Howard, Chelsea. Professor Armine Sefton and Michele Branscombe were also unwittingly invaluable in the preparation of this book by organising a fascinating and stimulating Master's course in Microbiology at Queen Mary University of London. Professors Graham Rook and Alimuddin Zumla of University College, London set me on the path of Infectious Diseases as a career, for which I thank them. Finally, I thank my family for their forbearance.

INTRODUCTION

The Quiet Killers?

Infectious diseases are very much on the minds of peoples and governments at present; we nervously anticipate the coming of a new pestilence in the form of epidemic avian influenza, or bird flu. Our hospitals are ridden with dangerous and untreatable bacteria. Each week seems to bring a new episode of food contamination. Whole industries in Britain have been brought to their knees by infections such as BSE and foot-and-mouth disease in cattle. Our antibiotics have stopped working. Could there be a more timely moment to publish a book about infectious diseases?

The title chosen for this book is 'Quiet Killers'. It concerns, as the subtitle explains, the fall and rise of infectious diseases. We should define precisely what we mean by that. We are concerned with those illnesses which are transmissible between people, from animals to people, from food, or in some cases from inanimate objects such as hospital equipment, and that have the power to cause death or severe disease. In some cases I have included transmissible agents which are less lethal than others, in order to make a more general point about the manner in which transmission may occur or illness result. The majority of the Quiet Killers are viruses or bacteria, but there are more complex and bizarre life forms, such as parasites and tape-worms, which fulfil our definition. One – the prion – seems barely to be a living thing at all, at least not by most useful definitions. We will proceed to examine why these may be considered 'quiet'. The adjective does not refer simply to their stealth. For some time infectious diseases have been considered quiet because we assumed they were receding. That assumption has proven to be wrong.

Let us take a moment to examine their power and danger. It is almost impossible to overstate the impact these diseases have had on human history. During the Great Plagues of history, the population of Europe was reduced by one third; the Black Death of 1348–9 may have killed half the population of Britain. We use the word 'decimate' to suggest massive destruction. The literal translation of decimate is to reduce by one tenth; it was the punishment meted out to rebellious legions of the Roman Empire. If decimate, then, means massive destruction with only 10 per cent mortality, what word would describe those plagues which killed 33 per cent of a whole continent?

Infectious diseases have been the major stalkers of man since history began. Although many historical records of death are inaccurate by modern standards (and our contemporary records may be so viewed in future), death by infection crops up again and again in parish records. Sometimes the cause of an infection has to be inferred from inexact medieval description – the 'Bloody Flux', for example, is what we would know as dysentery and 'Consumption' would almost certainly be tuberculosis (TB) – but without modern diagnostic methods many diseases, including cancer, would be indistinguishable. Causation of most diseases remained speculative until relatively recently. For example, the first suggestion that cholera might be an infectious agent transmitted through drinking water was raised by deduction. In 1849, John Snow, an anaesthetist from Yorkshire, suggested that material from human faeces might transmit the disease via improperly maintained sewers. It was many years before his hypothesis was proven, when the actual bacterium was isolated. Even as late as 1832, cholera was considered to be a divine visitation upon sinners.

Despite the inexact nature of historical records, we can make some estimate of the toll from diseases like the Plague, a toll which continues to this day. In the Great Plague of 1665 there were more than 68,000 recorded deaths in London alone. Rather like the current AIDS epidemic in Africa, mortality in the 'learned professions' was high. The Church suffered particularly severely. The economic and agricultural landscape of Europe was transformed forever. The last Great Plague epidemic began in 1894 and caused more than 100,000 deaths in Canton Province, China; in

1895, 1.3 million died in India. This epidemic is not quite over; there are still occasional cases and indeed deaths from the plague worldwide. The last case in Britain occurred in 1910.

The Government Register Office in England and Wales has systematically collected statistics on causes of death since 1837. The figures with respect to infectious disease make alarming reading both for the past and, for reasons I shall explain in the course of this book, for the future. It is not a straightforward task to compare years from these historical documents, because systems of classification of disease have changed and even the meanings of some of the words used have altered. For example, scarlet fever and diphtheria were not distinguished one from the other until 1855. Formal death registration by the doctor who saw the patient last was not introduced until 1874. For many years nebulous and vague causes of death such as 'old age', 'dropsy' and 'natural causes' were accepted by the Registrar; only in the latter half of the nineteenth century were more precise causes demanded. Nonetheless, broad conclusions may be drawn.

In the early days of the Government Register Office (1848–72), one death in three (321 per 1,000, to be exact) among males was ascribed to infectious disease. It should be noted that bronchitis and pneumonia – considered by most doctors to be at least in part due to infection – were counted separately. If they are included, then almost half of all deaths were due to infectious disease. Chief among these fatal infections – in Bunyan's phrase, 'Captain of the Men of Death' – was pulmonary tuberculosis (TB). One third of infectious disease deaths, or one ninth of all deaths, were due to TB, although pulmonary TB did not become a statutorily notifiable disease until 1911. Scarlet fever and diphtheria were next. The other major infectious killers were cholera, typhus, typhoid, influenza, measles, whooping cough and smallpox. By the time figures were collected between 1901 and 1910, the proportion of males dying from infectious disease had fallen to one in five; by 1981–5 the figure was 3 per 1,000. Cancer and heart disease have replaced infections as the major cause of death. Interestingly both may have an infectious component. However, it is only relatively recently that either (heart disease) has exceeded the historical mortality of TB.

The reasons for this decline in the importance of infectious diseases, and the possibility that the decline may be reversing, form much of the basis of this book. Many readers will be aware of the great publicity that has surrounded the emergence of resistant bacteria transmitted in hospitals – MRSA (methicillin-resistant *Staphylococcus* aureus) has achieved the greatest notoriety, although it is not the only bacterium or even the most dangerous. One organism, known as EMRAB (Epidemic Multi-Resistant *Acinetobacter baumanii*), has become resistant to just about every antibiotic in the pharmacy; there are other highly resistant organisms such as *Pseudomonas* spp. and *Burkholderia* spp. and, most worryingly, TB. There are, however, many further reasons for concern about the Quiet Killers and just what they are doing, lurking in the wings and gathering strength. This book charts the history of some of these killers and examines why in some cases they have fallen while in others they may now be rising again.

The bald figures of mortality, although they put the impact of infectious diseases into a numerical perspective, convey little of the human cost. A simple list of the great artists, poets, philosophers and politicians who are believed to have died of various infections – each of which might be cured nowadays – allows a less impersonal dimension. TB particularly has claimed so many famous lives that it deserves special mention. Here is a brief list of just some of the noted individuals who succumbed to 'consumption': Jane Austen, Honoré de Balzac, Anne Brontë, Charlotte Brontë, Emily Brontë, Charles Farrar Browne, Elizabeth Barrett Browning, Robert Burns, Anton Chekhov, Chopin (hideously, of massive pulmonary haemorrhage while seated at his piano), Stephen Crane, Jean de Brunhoff, Guy de Maupassant, Fyodor Dostoevsky, Éluard, Ralph Waldo Emerson, Maxim Gorky, Dashiell Hammett, Washington Irving, Samuel Johnson, Franz Kafka, John Keats, Charles Kingsley, D.H. Lawrence, Katherine Mansfield, Somerset Maugham, Molière, Eugene O'Neill, George Orwell, Edgar Allan Poe, Alexander Pope, Edmond Rostand, Jean-Jacques Rousseau, John Ruskin, Friedrich Schiller, Sir Walter Scott, Tobias Smollett, Laurence Sterne, Robert Louis Stevenson, Dylan Thomas, Francis Thompson, Henry David

Thoreau, Tut'ankhamun, Thomas Wolfe. How different the world might be had they survived – as they almost certainly would today.

The Quiet Killers have had colourful and epic consequences in history. One of my favourite anecdotes concerns Oliver Cromwell. I have family connections in Ireland, where his reputation is perhaps not quite as assured as it is elsewhere in the world, so this story has particular resonance for me. In 1658, Cromwell stood at the head of his powers. He had unseated one of Europe's oldest monarchies and replaced it with a republic, with himself at the head as Lord Protector. He had been swept to victory by the most efficient military machine of the age, the New Model Army. His combination of ruthless military efficiency and religious zealotry had proven unstoppable.

Then the wheels began to come off. In 1658, he fell ill with the 'tertian ague'. The method of diagnosis then was much the same as when Hippocrates first described it; in fact, descriptions of 'mal aria' (bad air) go back to 1000 BC – there is a characteristic fever on alternate days. Cromwell was a fensman, a farmer from the marshes of Lincolnshire. Before these marshes, or fens, were properly drained, malaria was endemic to this region and surrounding counties. It was also widespread on either side of the Thames Estuary in Essex and Kent; around the Bristol Channel; and around Romsey and Pevensey.

By 1640, the colonial Spanish had learned of a native remedy for malaria using the bitter bark of the 'fever tree' that grew in the montane rainforests along the eastern slopes of the northern Andes. The natives called it quinquina, the 'bark of barks'. Legend has it that the Count of Cinchon used it as a last resort to cure his wife's malaria, so the genus of the tree was named *Cinchona*. It was introduced into Rome by Spanish priests in 1632. First records of its use in England date from 1656. You might have thought that for Cromwell the cure was straightforward. However, he simply refused to take it.

The Catholic Jesuits had brought the bark back to Europe from Peru, a Portuguese colony. In the London Pharmacopoiea of 1677, it is recorded as *Cortex peruanus*. Cromwell's iron religious principles would not let him ingest a cure from a papist settlement;

'The Powder of the Devil', he called it. So Cromwell died of complications from malaria at Whitehall in the afternoon of 3 September 1658, aged 59 and victim of his own bigotry; a fitting end, many in Ireland might think.

His premature death left a hiatus in the transfer of power among the new hierarchy. Authority passed almost by default into the hands of Cromwell's son, Richard. His rule was so inept that he earned the nickname 'Tumbledown Dick'. The chaos that ensued paved the way for the Restoration of the Monarchy in 1688. Had Cromwell taken the Devil's Bark, then – who knows? – England might still be a republic.

There are a few inconvenient anomalies in this apocryphal anecdote. First, tertian ague, endemic to Britain in the seventeenth century, was and is seldom fatal. Fatal malaria is more usually caused by the parasite *Plasmodium falciparum*, which has never been established in the climate of northern Europe. Second, Cromwell's cause of death at the time was believed to be septicaemia from a urinary tract infection. Seventeenth-century medical science was inexact, but even then it would have been hard to confuse tertian ague with a urinary infection. Some believe that Cromwell was poisoned by his physician. Whatever the case, the fact that the anecdote has gained widespread acceptance testifies to the power of infectious diseases in folklore. Chaucer knew of malaria, as did Shakespeare, who refers to its horrors in *Henry V*: 'He is so shak'd of a burning quotidian that is most lamentable to behold' (*Henry V*, II: i: 123). Malaria has also been associated with the premature deaths or illnesses of St Augustine, King James I, King Charles II and Cardinal Wolsey. Alexander the Great may also have died of malaria (this is discussed in more detail below). There is another Cromwell anecdote later in the book: his bigotry may have been responsible for one of the greatest worldwide infectious disease epidemics of the eighteenth and nineteenth centuries; that being Yellow Fever.

Unsurprisingly, given the historical prevalence of infectious diseases, many other great names from history succumbed to or suffered from other contagions. Robert the Bruce almost certainly had leprosy, a condition widespread in Europe well into the Middle

Ages with occasional cases reintroduced from the Crusades. St James's Park in London is a former leper colony; St James is the patron saint of this bacterial disease. There was also a major leper colony at the ancient spa town of Bath. Gustav Mahler's tragic early death from infectious endocarditis is well documented. Roosevelt, although he eventually died of a cerebral haemorrhage, was greatly disabled during his life by childhood polio. Randolph Churchill, Winston's father, is believed by some to have died aged 45 from syphilis. In what state might the world be now had this infection been transmitted to his son in the womb? Congenital syphilis is often fatal to the embryo; surviving children may be grossly deformed and intellectually challenged. Something of a handicap in Winston Churchill's battle with Hitler, you might think.

In 323 BC, Alexander the Great stood at the head of the greatest empire the world had ever known. He had conquered the Persian Empire, including Anatolia, Syria, Phoenicia, Gaza, Egypt, Bactria and Mesopotamia, and extended the boundaries of his own empire as far as the Punjab. But then, aged 32, he fell ill with a fever in Babylon. The cause of his final illness is still debated. Among the infections suggested are West Nile Virus, typhoid and malaria. These last two are now curable; West Nile Virus not so. But had Alexander not died, had he lived even to 46 like his father, Philip of Macedon, where might the boundaries of his empire then be? It is, of course, possible that he did not die of an infection at all. Some believe he had alcoholic cirrhosis, while others say he was poisoned.

Henry VIII is a similar case. His cause of death is almost invariably cited as syphilis. His paranoia, rift with Rome, relentless and restless yet fruitless and subfertile search for a healthy male heir are often cited as evidence that he died of the Great Pox, as it was then known. It was so called to distinguish it from smallpox. Is it true that he died of syphilis? It is certainly true that paranoia is a feature of General Paresis of the Insane and that children born with congenital syphilis would be sickly, many dying young. Such was the fate of several of Henry's offspring. However, for reasons outlined above, we shall never know. The diagnosis of syphilis has only lately become a relatively exact science. Wassermann's first test for syphilis – the VDRL test – was only described in 1899, some 400 years after Henry Tudor died. Some say he died of gout; others from delayed consequences of a jousting injury. An image contained within his own prayer book, however, is said to show syphilitic damage to his nose.

The political effects of infectious diseases are not solely confined to those famous names who have succumbed to them. Whole economies and agricultural systems have fallen and risen as the consequence of plagues and pestilences. Military campaigns have been jeopardized, wars lost and won by the Quiet Killers. Apart from biological warfare (which will be considered later in more detail), infections have been the scourge of armies since 'civilisation' required them to be raised. In the Crimean War, for example, infectious disease accounted for far more lives lost than enemy action. It was this campaign which inspired Florence Nightingale in her efforts to reform the care of injured and sick soldiers; her efforts (however misguided) to control infection systematically were to transform healthcare for ever. In the Boer War of 1901–3, typhoid infected 105 of every 1,000 soldiers; by the time of the First World War, when inoculation of soldiers was routine, the figure had fallen to 2.35 per 1,000.

That war – the First World War – is often regarded as the apogee of senseless slaughter; a testament to the folly of humankind and a sort of low watermark of civilisation. Yet infectious disease in the form of influenza, a disease we have until recently regarded as not much more than an inconvenience, caused more deaths in the period immediately following the Armistice than the First and Second World Wars combined. We have every reason now to fear that such 'inconvenience' might again trouble us on a similar scale. Avian influenza, to which humans have no natural immunity, has killed scores of people at the time of writing; has mutated into a more dangerous form; and has crossed the gates of Europe. An outbreak in Nigeria looks to be uncontrolled. Whether or not this will develop into the next major Quiet Killer remains to be seen. It is salutary that some believe that the Great Influenza Pandemic of 1918 began as bird flu. It was inoculated into soldiers foraging for

8

migratory birds in a war-ravaged continent, who then disseminated the infection across the globe on demobilisation.

The continuing impact of infectious diseases is not simply due to their mortality. These diseases can be highly debilitating. Consider tapeworm infections. You may not have thought of these as infectious diseases; however, they are living organisms that are transmitted through food, the skin or the bite of an insect, and cause massive burden of illness throughout the world. Many may be treated by simple, harmless tablets. Several studies have shown that African children given a drug called levamisole – irrespective of whether or not they are shown to be infected with tapeworms – grow 5 per cent taller and even, in one study, show a significant improvement in academic performance following a single treatment with the drug. In an act of magnificent generosity, the inventor of another drug active against parasites, called ivermectin, has given it to the world absolutely free; this will be discussed later in greater detail.

Other infectious diseases remain dreadful scourges of the developing world. To an extent these are Quiet Killers not because they make no noise, but because nobody is listening. Those dry, dusty figures from history become uncomfortably relevant to the modern day when you start counting deaths from infectious diseases in the current Third World. Consider malaria, the killer of Byron. At present, malaria kills one person every 30 seconds, many of these children. It killed more people in the twentieth century than both World Wars. It affects five times as many people as TB, AIDS, leprosy and measles combined. There is no really effective vaccine, and resistance to anti-malarial drugs is an almost insurmountable problem (this is discussed in more detail in Chapter Three). Even simple infectious diarrhoea causes millions of deaths in places where there is no reliable clean water supply and no access to even basic medical care. Typhoid, TB and plague still kill. Readily preventable and treatable infectious conditions such as chlamydia cause blindness for millions worldwide. Polio, once a major cause of disability in the western world, has been more or less eradicated in the West but is showing worrying signs of recurrence in Africa.

Finally, AIDS today ravages entire continents, skewing the demographics of whole nations and leaving millions orphaned.

What would have happened if all the millions who died of infectious diseases had not done so? It is possible, of course, that we would have a massively overpopulated planet. Some say that we already do, and our control of infectious diseases has of course contributed to that. But a feature of overcrowding and overpopulation is increased susceptibility to disease, particularly diseases of infection. Some might hypothesise a natural, Gaia-like symmetry in this state of affairs: populations and diseases occur in balance. When numbers increase to unsustainable levels, then there is a natural cull. I have heard this argument put forward by at least one eminent physician. When a colleague presented his work that was leading to the development of the elusive vaccine for TB, he was asked who would then look after all the people who survived?

I find this point of view distasteful. First, the evidence is that Malthus – who proposed that populations unchecked would grow to unsustainable numbers – was wrong. The birth rate of educated, healthy populations free of infectious diseases tends to fall, not rise. Healthy populations are more capable of managing their own affairs than diseased ones. As we will see in Chapter Eleven, humankind is a clever animal: we can usually find ways of averting famine and drought, but more easily when these are not accompanied by the other pestilences, war and disease, and the fifth pestilence – indifference.

*   *   *

It is easy to draw the conclusion that diseases of infection are exclusively malign. As will be discussed in greater detail in Chapter Six, this may not be the whole truth. First, we would probably not be as we are without the evolutionary challenge of infectious disease. Second, the definition of what constitutes an infection is almost arbitrary: our bodies play host to billions of organisms which could easily kill us in the right circumstances. Some infections are like garden weeds: there is nothing intrinsically wrong with the plant, but it just happens to be in the wrong place. The bacteria we harbour – and in at least one case, a virus – actually do us a great deal of good. Some microbiologists argue that we are essentially composed of microbes, living in huge communities with the emergent properties of life and consciousness. Finally, there is increasing evidence that we have erred in trying to protect ourselves from infection; some 'infections' may be highly beneficial to us.

This book will discuss the nature of the Quiet Killers from a number of angles that I hope will give insight into their nature and the problems they cause; their past history; and our future alongside them. In the first chapter, I will discuss those diseases that appear to have gone away: smallpox, polio, diphtheria, plague, the 'Bloody Flux' and scarlatina. Have they really gone? Why? Could they come back? What were they like? I then discuss the ones that are coming back, or are changing their distribution. These include malaria, TB, syphilis, gonorrhoea and rabies. Could malaria return to haunt us in the West? Is the progress of rabies across Europe unstoppable? Later chapters discuss diseases that have remained with us over centuries; diseases that have spread in conditions of war and famine; new diseases; and diseases with the potential to kill us all.

Infectious diseases are 'Quiet Killers' for many different reasons, and the disparity between developed and undeveloped nations is the most telling. This is the silence of the proverbial tree falling in the forest – no one is listening. The book's title has been chosen for many other reasons, however. As we will discuss in the chapters on bioterrorism, untreatable infections and horrible rarities, there is something peculiarly visceral in our distaste for illness caused by microbes. Other methods of death – war, for example – have acquired an aura almost of kudos and glory, although this probably is not reflected in the experience of those who are actually involved. Other means of death may even allow us some wry amusement. One of my favourite short stories, by Graham Greene, concerns the son of a man who is killed by a pig falling from a balcony. The son's life is blighted by the fact that everyone to whom he tells the tragic tale cannot help laughing. Eventually he finds love, when he meets a woman who does not laugh. But there is no such dry entertainment to be found in the stealthy stalking of the Quiet Killers.

The title of this book has been chosen for other reasons too. The kind of person who likes to see cause and planning in the world would soon conclude that the Quiet Killers, the bugs that cause fatal infections, were designed by someone very clever indeed. For these bugs have evolved often sophisticated mechanisms and behaviours which enable them to evade the surveillance of our immunity. Like commandos, they sneak under the searchlights and cause death and illness. It is in this sense that they are 'quiet'. Like assassins, they creep up on us using artful means. This book is their story, and describes some of the mechanisms by which they invade.

Consider, for example, the parasite that causes sleeping sickness, an often fatal infection transmitted by biting flies in Africa. It wears a specialised coat made of a mixture of sugars and proteins. After the first infection, animal immune systems recognise these 'glycoproteins' and recruit deadly white blood cells to destroy the invader. Yet, just as the animal's immune system has processed all the data and is launching its first deadly assault on the enemy, *Trypanosoma brucei*, our sleeping sickness bug, slips off its glycoprotein overcoat and slips on a new one. It's just like something from a John le Carré novel. The parasite has a series of brilliant disguises which it dons in turn. Eventually, the immune system gives up and the poor victim becomes riddled with parasites, including in the brain, and dies.

Rabies is another example of combat by stealth. Caused by a virus, which is transmitted most commonly from the infected bites of warm-blooded animals, the infection may lie dormant for months to years after a bite. It migrates up through nerve tissue, gradually creeping towards the head. It moves slowly – about 1mm per day – but with direction and unstoppable determination. Once rabies causes symptoms, it is almost always (in more than 99 per cent of cases) fatal. When it finally reaches its destinations – the brain and the mouth – it has two simultaneous actions. The first is to reproduce in the salivary glands, so that the bite becomes infectious. The second is to inflame the brain, but in such a specific way that it makes the victim want to bite someone.

Let's just think about that for a moment. How big is the rabies virus? As viruses go, it's actually quite large, being about 400 nanometres long by about 100 nanometres in diameter. A nanometre is a billionth of a metre. If you are of average size, that means that you are about 400 million times as tall as the rabies virus. If you are of average height, I am probably slightly taller than you, by a few centimetres. What would I have to do to get you to bite someone – possibly a friend or relation – in order to get you to transmit a fatal disease? I would have to be very persuasive indeed, or be very powerful, or carry some sort of weapon. Even then most of you would probably refuse. Microbes can do things that we just can't, and across unimaginable differences of scale.

How could the astonishing faculties of these tiny life forms have arisen? Does rabies, a virus only visible under the electron microscope, do its brilliant trick of changing the behaviour of a human many billions of times its own mass because God made it do so? Or because it has evolved into performing the task over millennia, simply to ensure its own survival and transmission? Whether you believe that the astounding complexity of micro-organisms has arisen by creation and a divine purpose, or was cooked up by the Devil, or has arisen by Darwinian natural selection, makes no difference. These observations about microbes are, I think, cause for the same awe and wonder whatever you believe. They tell us about the miraculous diversity of the world in which we live; and they reflect our own complexity and diversity. There would be no point in *Trypanosoma brucei* performing its Master of Disguise trick if our immune systems were not so sophisticated and adaptable; the two of course evolved together.

Understanding of the mechanisms by which microbes survive and flourish is more than just a diverting parlour game for the scientifically curious. It has been detailed examination of their behaviour which has allowed us to intercede and kill or suppress them, and moreover to understand why we seem to be losing the war against them. Fleming's discovery of penicillin, the seminal moment in modern treatment of infection, relied on the way that bacteria need a tough cell wall to survive and multiply in a hostile world. Bacteria have a problem with scale: they have a large surface to area ratio, and are therefore prone to drying out and dying. They also have contents which are under pressure – *Staphylococcus aureus* has an internal pressure about fifty times that of Earth's atmosphere. Without the 'string bag' of the cell wall, the bacteria simply pop. If you observe a staphylococcus after treatment with penicillin, you'll see that's exactly what it does.

Our cells don't need that cell wall. Thus drugs which target it are, generally, harmless to us unless we are allergic to them. Looking in detail at the structure of the string bag of bacteria has allowed us to develop some of the most useful antibiotics and antimicrobials in our pharmacies. This is one of many ways in which exploiting the differences between the way that microbes and animal cells behave has allowed us to develop other useful drugs. Just as important, and more exciting, is the way the bugs have 'learned' to evade the drugs. It is these unexpected properties which today pose science some of its greatest challenges.

The quest to contain and destroy the Quiet Killers could not have begun without knowledge of how cells work. The key to life, the ultimate structure of what makes us, was, I believe, initially discovered not by Watson and Crick in their famous crystal-snapshots of DNA, but by the amazing and radical discovery of a microbiologist called Fred Griffiths. There has always been some dispute about whether Watson and Crick deserved their Nobel Prizes in preference to others involved in the discovery of DNA. There is no doubt in my mind that Griffiths deserved it more than either of them.

Fred Griffiths was a microbiologist with an interest in *Streptococcus pneumoniae*, the bacterium that commonly causes pneumonia, as its name suggests. It is not restricted to causing pneumonia, but we will let that pass for a moment. In 1928, Griffiths performed a series of experiments which were to transform science, and as if to emphasise that fact the principle he discovered was called transformation. He knew that there were two forms of the bacterium, rough and smooth mutants. They were so called because of their physical appearance on the agar plate. The difference was due to a complex sugar contained in the coat of the bacterium. This sugar is vital to the bacterium in identifying and invading its targets. Unlike their harmless rough cousins, the smooth mutants were rapidly lethal when injected into mice. Griffiths killed the lethal smooth mutants and then allowed their corpses to mingle with colonies of the living, harmless rough ones. These promptly became smooth, *and became lethal.* In other words, like some disarmed soldiers that come across a slaughtered army they were able to loot weapons for their own purposes. From this moment forward, the scientific quest was to identify the structure of what began to be called the genetic code. Its existence could not be in any doubt. It is hard to think of any simple experiment which has altered our perception of life as much as this one. Griffiths himself exits the story at this point. In 1944, Avery, MacLeod and McCarty unravelled the transforming principle. It was DNA.

*   *   *

Let us take a step back to Fleming's discovery of penicillin. Penicillin is famously produced by a naturally occurring fungus. It is believed to have drifted in through Fleming's window from the Fountains Abbey pub opposite. The pub and Fleming's lab are both still open, the latter as a museum. Within a very few months, Fleming observed that some bacteria were resistant to his fungal extract. He had previously noted that some sorts of bugs were 'inherently' resistant to penicillin; many have the wrong kind of 'string bag' for penicillin to be active. However, he soon realised that the type of bugs which initially responded to penicillin sometimes lost their responsiveness in time.

If you ask most doctors how it is that bacteria acquire resistance to antibiotics, they will reply, 'mutation'. The truth is, in fact, far more interesting than simple random accidents in the genetic code of our enemies. Within a very short space of time, Fleming was able to find bacteria which had acquired resistance. Remember that this was resistance to a naturally occurring substance produced by a naturally occurring fungus. This works because the bacteria, having found themselves under attack, are able to produce a chemical, an enzyme called beta-lactamase, that specifically damages the structure of the penicillin molecule.

Enzymes are complex molecules, usually made of many amino acids. Each amino acid requires its own bit of DNA to code for it. Bacteria reproduce very rapidly, and there are huge numbers of them in a colony. Bacterial DNA is more prone to mutation than animal DNA. Even so, the chances of a sufficient number of mutations accumulating such that the bacteria were able to produce anything as complex as an entirely new enzyme are vanishingly small. But there is another, simpler explanation.

Supposing you were being chased down a hotel corridor by a mad axeman. There are hundreds of doors to choose from. You have a key in your pocket. What gives you the best chance of survival? Knowing which door to unlock, of course. Your chances of survival are massively increased if you have been down that corridor before. So it is with *Staphylococci*. The bacteria had met the fungus and its armoury before.

As the fungus and the bacteria co-evolved, they would have competed for niches in the environment. For a while the bacteria might have had the upper hand, and then the fungi, and then the bacteria again in an increasingly complex and sophisticated struggle. The fungi have eventually come up with antibiotics, tiny little balloons that interfere with string bag production. Then the bacteria came up with the beta-lactamase to destroy those antibiotics. In fact, the beta-lactamase enzyme that the bacteria use to destroy penicillin is really just a modified version of the enzyme they use to produce their own string bag. The bacteria need a sort of knitting-needle to produce their string bags, and beta-lactamase is a bit like a sharpened knitting-needle. The situation becomes more complex, as discussed below, when we look at how bacteria are capable of sharing their sharpened knitting-needles, even across species.

This may seem to labour the point rather. However, this story reveals several key facts about the Quiet Killers. First, dangerous infectious bugs have not evolved in isolation. Most have been around for far longer than we have, and they have seen it all before. Second, they compete with one another to live in specialised niches in the environment, and to do so they produce weapons to fight one another. Some of these weapons are dangerous to humans. The fact that they cause disease in humans is probably accidental in many cases. Third, because the adaptations produced by competition for survival are ongoing, no matter how carefully we scour the world for substances that kill bacteria and viruses, eventually we are going to lose the battle.

There is another, perhaps even more unexpected, aspect to microbe behaviour, and that is the fact that as they live in social 'communities' these bugs can 'learn' from and adapt to each other. When most of us think of bugs that cause disease, we think either of the disease itself or of colonies of bugs happily reproducing in petri dishes in the laboratory. For years, scientists have derived their conclusions about bacteria from observations of their behaviour in these artificial laboratory environments. Lately, microbiologists have discovered that bugs are a whole load more interesting than that. Would it surprise you to learn that bacteria live, often harmoniously, in multiracial communities? That they talk to each other? Hold board meetings to decide on plans of action? Feed each other? Fight each other? Protect each other? Sleep? Share news and information? Pass on tips for fighting antibiotics? They even talk to you, and you talk back to them. Each of us is in fact in a state of continuous conversation with the bacteria that share our lives, determining whether we live in a state of truce or war.

Looked at in its simplest form, bugs share information in the crudest way by competing for nutrients and ecological niches. You could argue that this isn't really communication, but just Darwinian competition. However, if you look back at the example above, where fungi and bacteria were competing and evolving alongside each other, you'd be hard put to say precisely what the difference was between this and communication. The difference was that the communication took the form of an argument. The fungi and bacteria exchanged information, albeit hostile, that was of ultimate benefit to both. If that isn't communication, I don't know what is. Perhaps the Quiet Killers are not quite so silent after all.

Not all bacteria interact in a competitive way. Some feed one another, passing on waste products that are nutritious to other species. There are advantages to both here: excessive accumulation of waste products is as toxic to bacteria as it is to us. Enormously complex communities of bacteria can build up in this way. Each species will have its own function. Some species – *Staphylococci*, for example – are very good at anchoring to inert material and producing dense slime that other bacteria can stick to. *Streptococci* are marvellous at absorbing genes, processing them and passing them on to other bacteria. Both of these bacteria consume oxygen, which allows pockets of oxygen-starved environment to form. In those pockets, bacteria that can only live in oxygen-deprived conditions will thrive; these are the anaerobes.

These communities are called biofilms, and most of us are familiar with them already, even though you may not know it. You brush biofilms off your teeth every morning and night. Biofilms cause food spoilage in factories; taint beer in breweries; and slow down ships on the sea by sticking to their hulls. If you have ever applied anti-foul to the hull of a boat, you have tried to prevent a biofilm forming.

This is of more than just academic and industrial interest. The biofilm in your mouth is responsible for what many believe is the commonest infectious disease in the world – tooth decay. Bacteria in the biofilm produce acid, which damages the tough enamel of your teeth. In doing so, it provides a rougher, more hospitable surface for bacteria to thrive, and releases nutrients. Unchecked, it will mean a trip to the dentist for you. Biofilms also stick to plumbing pipes in houses and hotels. This has allowed one of the newer killers of recent years to emerge. *Legionella pneumophila*, the agent of fatal Legionnaires' disease, cannot survive very well in an inert environment. However, give it a nice warm biofilm full of bugs and it will thrive. Deadly *Legionella* may be cultured from 10 per cent of domestic hot water systems. We will meet *Legionella* again later.

You probably don't find it all that surprising that bacteria can share nutrients and live in communities. The other ways in which bacteria can communicate are far more unexpected. The first intimation that bacteria could talk to one another was discovered in the 1970s, and in the most unlikely of places – squid eyes. Certain species of squid and fish use bacteria for a specific purpose. Colonies of a marine bacterium called *Vibrio fischeri* inhabit their eye sockets. *Vibrio fischeri* has a particular property that is useful to the squid and the fish: it glows. This provides a sort of set of headlights for the squid, so it can detect prey, and scares away predators. Of course, a single bacterium would be of very little use to the squid as it would not generate enough light, so whole colonies of millions of bacteria have to form to line the eye sockets.

Marine biologists observing the bacteria in cultures noted that they had a startling property. A single bacterium did not glow. Nor did ten. Or a thousand. Or a million. Only when a certain critical number threshold was reached did the bacteria start to glow. The explanation for this seems obvious enough – there isn't much point in a single bacterium wasting energy glowing as it wouldn't help the squid or the bacterium and it would die of exhaustion. The interesting question was, how did each bacterium know when to start glowing?

The scientists investigating this phenomenon took their tests a stage further. They allowed a flask of *Vibrios* to glow until they were exhausted. They then centrifuged the colony to separate the bacteria from the fluid they were living in. They than added the fluid to a new flask of fresh *Vibrio fischeri* that were not glowing. And . . . they started to glow.

In other words, the bacteria were producing some sort of signal to each other. The signal was to let one another know when there were enough of them present to make it worth their while glowing. The scientists purified the signal present in the solution, and found it to be a chemical called homoserine lactone. The signal depended on there being enough bacteria producing enough homoserine lactone to switch the lights on. For this reason – that a 'quorum' was needed, just as in a board meeting – this was named quorum sensing.

For years, quorum sensing was ignored as an interesting oddity, little more. More recently, though, it has begun to dawn on us that many, many bacteria use quorum sensing for various purposes. Some bacteria – *Pseudomonas aeruginosa*, for example – will only start producing poisonous substances if there are enough of them present to make it worthwhile, rather like an army waiting till the troops are all lined up. And it is this ability to save their energies, thus making them invisible to the host while congregating in their masses before making a deadly assault, that makes some of our Quiet Killers so dangerous.

It is just this sort of extraordinary and enthralling cunning and the danger of these organisms that has informed the creation of this book. Before progressing any further, I should clarify one or two issues. This is not a textbook. It is in no way intended to be a complete account of all infectious diseases that afflict humankind. Any medical student or nurse hoping to use it to help pass an examination will most certainly fail unless they use other sources. Nor is it a vade mecum or encyclopaedia for those concerned about infection. What I have sought to do is simply include the aspects of infectious diseases that have interested me in the hope that they will interest you. I have also used a system of exploring these fascinating life forms that would be anathema to any editor of a textbook, being whimsical and unsystematic. I have read many textbooks and contributed to several. I do not think you would thank me for offering another. I have no doubt that medically trained readers and reviewers will point to glaring omissions; I make no apology. I have simply included those diseases, or aspects of diseases, that I find absorbing. Overall, I hope you will gain some insight into the fascinating world of dangerous infectious organisms. I hope you will share some of my enthusiasm for the diseases to which I have devoted my professional life. These organisms are no more or less adapted to their environment, no less a miracle of creation, than any other life form on the planet. One could almost grow to love them, if only they didn't kill us.

ONE

Dead and Gone?
Diseases that have gone away

What is the Bloody Flux, anyway? Why doesn't anyone die of it any more? Or dropsy, for that matter. Should we care? When I think of the disappearance of once common scourges like the Bloody Flux, I am reminded of those incomplete medieval maps which plotted all that was known up to the edge of the explored world. In some of the maps you might find a fantastic sea-creature depicted, bobbing about in the waves, with the caption, 'Here Be Monsters'. Not only have we filled in beyond the boundaries of the map, but we also know the nature of the monsters. They are sharks of course, or (on land) crocodiles, or other potentially man-eating but commonplace beasts. Knowing what they are makes them no less dangerous, but their classification has taken away some of their terror. We also know how to avoid them; as mankind encroaches ever further into the wilder reaches of the planet and steals their habitat they further lose their menace.

So it has been with these diseases. The flux is an abnormally copious flowing of blood, excrement from the bowels or any organ; a morbid or excessive discharge. Thus it was an early term for dysentery. The first recorded use of the term is in Wycliff's bible of 1382: 'A womman that soffride the flix, or rennynge, of blood twelve yeer.' The association with blood implies either amoebic or bacillary dysentery, usually caused by the protozoan amoeba *Entamoeba hystolytica*; or bacteria, principally of the *Shigella* and *E. coli* groups.

Of course people do still die of dysentery, but rarely in the developed world. Special circumstances generally apply. Patients severely debilitated by advanced AIDS or cancer may sometimes succumb to it. There are some inherited defects of immunity that might lead to children and babies suffering incurable bloody diarrhoea. Severe and fatal diarrhoea caused by antibiotics – pseudomembranous colitis – may sometimes be bloody. The notorious *E. coli* 0157 may sometimes cause death with copious bloody stools even among healthy people. Fortunately, these are all fairly rare. However, in the developing world diarrhoeal illnesses remain one of the leading causes of death, especially among children.

The reasons that the Bloody Flux no longer kills in the West give fascinating insights into the nature of the Quiet Killers. The first and most obvious reason is that its name was simply changed. The Victorian era saw a massive and explosive development of our knowledge and understanding of infectious diseases. Right up until the middle of the nineteenth century, it was widely believed that such diseases as the Flux or cholera were punishments from God. The 'germ' hypothesis of disease was often scoffed at. When Robert Koch ended his lecture first demonstrating the world's most dangerous bacterium (the one that causes TB) on 24 March 1882, there was complete silence. No questions, no congratulations, no applause. The audience was too stunned to respond. Koch had to bring virtually his entire laboratory to the lecture theatre to prove his point.

And yet the existence of microbes had been known since the mid-seventeenth century. The Englishman Robert Hooke had been the first to describe them in 1665, by chance at about the time that the last Great Plagues were ravaging Europe. His microscopes were of relatively low magnification. The milling of lenses was then in its infancy, was performed by hand, and did not allow the visualisation of organisms much smaller than fungi. Yet he hypothesised that these tiny cellules were living things, an observation as remarkable for its time as the splitting of the atom.

Hooke's baton was taken up by the Dutchman Anton van Leeuwenhoek, a cloth merchant living in Delft. Van Leeuwenhoek was a thorough merchant in his business dealings. He liked to examine the warp and weft of fabrics under a magnifying glass before committing to purchase; only the finest textiles would satisfy him. By chance he visited England in 1668, and was amazed at the images available of magnified cloth fibres. Nothing in Holland could match it. He immediately headed home, determined to better the technology of the English lenses.

A painstaking man, Van Leeuwenhoek carefully worked at his lenses until he was able to achieve magnifications of 300–500 fold. He was lucky in having naturally fine vision, but even so the discriminatory powers of his simple machines (by 'simple' is meant a single lens, rather than a complex series of lenses as in modern microscopes) were astonishing for their time. He experimented with microscopes of silver and gold (for which reason they do not survive, as they were sold by his heirs), then used the world around him to test the resolution of his machines. He examined his own dental plaque, his own semen, and just about any fluid or substance that came across his path. He saw – and drew – tiny moving objects apparently going about their business in a purposeful manner; conspicuously alive.

He wrote to the Royal Society of London in 1676, and included drawings of his observations. His claim that these tiny moving shapes were animate, living beings caused shock and disbelief. However, even a brief visit to inspect the evidence of his microscopes was enough to convince the most sceptical of his critics. He became celebrated throughout Europe, demonstrating his 'animalcules' to the Great and the Good, including Tsar Feodor III of Russia.

With the benefit of the 'retrospectoscope', it is hard to comprehend how the link between these microbes and disease was not made. It was another 200 years before the link between bacteria and disease was incontrovertibly established. Partly, this was due to the character of Van Leeuwenhoek himself. His fastidious and meticulous nature meant that he refused to permit anyone to handle his microscopes; he would prepare the experiment himself and simply allow the viewer to peer down the lens. This treatment was meted out to everyone, be they the Tsar of all the Russias or his own next-door neighbour. However, the notion that diseases were caused by living creatures was almost impossible for scientists of the seventeenth century to comprehend, as it meant rejecting orthodoxies built up over centuries.

Nevertheless, it had been understood since the earliest times that diseases could be transmitted from person to person; it was just that nobody knew how. During outbreaks of plague and smallpox, many fled before the advancing scourges; sometimes whole villages were abandoned. The bizarre 'plague masks' (sometimes in the shape of animals or birds) worn in medieval cities are testament to the theory of contagion of the time. The quarantining of ships in harbour to prevent the introduction of diseases such as Yellow Fever was introduced long before the transmissible agent was identified. The isolation of lepers in closed colonies to reduce transmission is an ancient tradition which persists even today.

As we have said, the nature of the infectious agent was frequently mistaken. Malaria derives its name from the Italian 'mal aria', or bad air. For many years, it was believed that noxious vapours arising from marshland were the cause of the febrile illness. The plague was also believed to be transmitted through the air, by evil spirits; such spirits could be deterred by certain herbs, or masks, or flowers. How these evil spirits caused disease was never really questioned; indeed, the origins of any kind of life were shrouded in a fallacious but surprisingly tenacious theory that persisted almost until the modern age: spontaneous generation.

Several key scientists challenged the commonly held view of the nature of infection in the years between Van Leeuwenhoek's amazing discovery and the modern age. For many hundreds of years, it was believed that some kinds of infection – lice, maggots and beetles – arose by spontaneous generation. The origin of life itself was believed to be just that: life arising naturally from a combination of heat, light, moisture and non-living matter. Horseflies, for example, transmuted from rotting manure.

Francesco Redi, a seventeenth-century scholar, biologist, physician and Renaissance man, who also established the mode of action of snake venom, refuted the theory of spontaneous generation by a simple and elegant experiment. He placed meat in jars. One jar was left open, another sealed with cork, and another shielded with fine netting. Predictably to us, but to the astonishment of thinkers of the day, only the meat open to the air (and, as we now know,

24

contamination by flies) developed maggots. Paradoxically, Van Leeuwenhoek's animalculi briefly breathed life back into the spontaneous generation fallacy; indeed, the theory refused to die out fully for many years to come. Some scientists, notably the Frenchmen Pouchet and Bastian, were still championing it at the end of the nineteenth century. The problem was that every apparently watertight challenge to the theory of spontaneous generation was held to have flaws. Spallanzini showed that microbes did not appear in heated, sealed flasks, but did in unheated and unsealed ones. Ah!, said the devotees of spontaneous generation, heating spoils the air in which the process might occur! Gradually, by improving the sophistication of the experiments to counter each challenge from the shrinking number of true believers in the traditional theory, spontaneous generation began to look increasingly shaky. Chief among the scientists responsible for this were Schröder, Tyndall and Louis Pasteur.

Pasteur decided to settle the vexed question of spontaneous generation once and for all in 1859. His famous experiment was brilliantly simple. He placed boiled, sterile broth in long-necked glass flasks. He then drew out the necks of the flask, so that they still contained unheated air and were open to the world, but only via a curved route. He believed that contaminating microbes would sediment into the shallow u-bend formed by the curved neck of the flasks. His broths remained uncontaminated even when observed for months – unless he tipped the flask so that the broth came into contact with the curved neck, where the microbes from the air had landed. He also unravelled another source of failure of some experiments devoted to spontaneous generation: some bacteria formed spores, which were highly resistant to sterilisation by boiling. These experiments, which could easily be repeated by other scientists, finally and completely annihilated the theory of spontaneous generation.

Then, some doctors – most famously, a Yorkshire anaesthetist called John Snow – began to hypothesise that, for instance, cholera might be transmitted by sewage-contaminated water. Snow's theory was based on observations that certain houses in London's Soho were affected during an epidemic of cholera, whereas others were not. He speculated that the houses where people had the illness drew their water from a particular pump. The handle of the pump, on Broad Street (now called Broadwick Street) was removed – sadly, shortly after the epidemic had naturally ended. There is a plaque commemorating Snow's achievement at the site of the pump, next to a pub that also bears his name. The natural conclusion from his observations was that an infectious agent was responsible. It was fifty years before Koch – he of the tubercle bacillus – identified the organism.

Why was Koch able to identify the cholera organism, when microscopes capable of visualising bacteria had been available since the mid-seventeenth century? The development of microbiology as a discipline really only began in the late nineteenth century. Strangely enough, the greatest advances were by-products of the textile industry and of simple housewifery.

Industrial processes of mass production in the second half of the nineteenth century demanded cheap and plentiful replacements for the natural dyes (cochineal, purples from coral and so on) that had been used for centuries. Mill owners turned to the chemists for new sources of dyes; and modern fashions also demanded brighter, more vivid and more durable colours. These dyes had qualities that made them ideal for the developing medical sciences. They penetrated and adhered to living – or recently deceased – tissue. They stained different kinds of material in different ways. In the field of histopathology, for example, certain kinds of cell stained in dramatically different colours from others. For the first time, it was possible to discriminate between different kinds of white blood cell; and even to visualise cancer cells. Up until this point tissue preparations were traditionally stained with one of the so-called natural dyes such as carmine or saffron. The first aniline dye, for textile staining, was produced by Perkin in 1856. This transformed the choice of dye for laboratory purposes. Significant new techniques followed: the 'H&E' in the period 1875–8, and the 'Ziehl Neilsson' for tubercle bacilli in 1883. The famous Gram stain was developed in 1884. Other stains followed rapidly – Giemsa, Romanowsky, Warthin-Starry.

Now we must meet a man to whom the world, and not just the world of medicine, owes an enormous debt of gratitude. He straddled the disciplines of medicine – microbiology, pathology, immunology, pharmacology – like a colossus, in a way which only now is again at the very forefront of medical science, but was then unheard of. His name was Paul Ehrlich. He was born on 14 March 1854, in Strehlen, Silesia, Prussia (now Strzelin, Poland). His family were prosperous, and able to support the young Ehrlich's precocious fascination with chemistry. Even in childhood, he would pester the town's chemist with prescriptions of his own devising. He qualified in medicine in 1878, and subsequently worked in the laboratory of his friend Robert Koch. Almost casually, he invented the science of histopathology. Other doctors would examine whole body parts post-mortem for evidence of disease; Ehrlich had the brilliant idea of paring organs into wafer-thin, translucent sections, which he then dyed with the new aniline stains and observed down the microscope.

He noted the presence of bacteria in some of his tissue slices. He recognised a phenomenon that was to transform the way we treat infections; and indeed other diseases such as cancers and immunological conditions. What he noticed was that certain dyes adhered to certain animal and human tissues, while other cells rejected them. Further, certain parts of the cells would accept the dyes while others would not. Exactly the same applied to bacteria, protozoa and the whole range of micro-organisms that caused human diseases.

Now, for the first time, it was possible to identify the bugs which caused disease by their differential staining. For example, the bacteria that cause TB do not absorb Gram's stain; TB bacilli will therefore not be visible when tissue from a TB abscess is stained with those chemicals. However, stain the same tissue with the Ziehl Neilsson stain and hey presto! – there is your bug. It seems so obvious now.

Throughout the 1890s, Ehrlich carried out important work in immunology. The value of his research was recognised, and in 1899 he became Director of the Royal Institute of Experimental Therapy in Frankfurt. In 1908, he received the Nobel Prize for Medicine for his work in immunology.

Simple domestic advice from a housewife made possible a further enormous stride in the development of microbiology as a science. Walter Hesse was a German family doctor who had an interest in public health and the metabolism of bacteria. In 1881, he obtained a post in the laboratory of the same Robert Koch. Koch and his colleagues had a particular problem one summer. They used to try to grow the bacteria they wished to examine on petri dishes containing solidified gelatine. Walter Hesse had special difficulty with the plates he was using to count the number of contaminating bacteria in air samples. The gelatine consistently melted, and was then digested by the bacteria. Hesse asked his wife – born Fanny Angelina Eilshemius, but known as Lina – how she managed to keep her jellies and puddings solid in the hot weather. Lina replied that she used agar-agar, a seaweed extract. Lina had lived as a child in New York, next to a family of Dutch immigrants who had been living in Java. Of Dutch ancestry herself, Lina had spent much time with them, and had learnt about agar-agar from them; it had been used as a gelling agent in the Far East for centuries.

Hesse tested the complex sugar polysaccharide seaweed extract as a supporting medium for his bacterial colonies and found that it worked to perfection. It didn't kill the bugs; it didn't kill him; it stayed solid even in the greatest summer heat; it didn't mind being sterilised at 100°C and above; and as it was a complex sugar, most bacteria were unable to digest it. This simple household item allowed doctors to inspect the lives of the Quiet Killers in a detail that had never before been possible. Previously, isolating and culturing bacteria on solid media had been laborious and demanding; now, a technician with the most basic training could achieve it. As it happens, some of the most interesting behaviour of bacteria is lost when they are trapped in the pure and – by bacterial standards – sterile world of the agar petri dish. Their ability to talk to each other, to fight, to live as communities in peace and harmony – all of these are lost when they live in pure colonies on agar. Nonetheless, modern microbiology really began at this moment.

New techniques, based on genetic fingerprinting of bacteria, are being developed all the time. Yet almost every microbiology laboratory in the world continues to use good old Frau Hesse's agar-agar as the basic medium for growing bacteria, as well as the stains devised by Gram, Ehrlich and Giemsa.

So many great advances against the Quiet Killers were made in Koch's laboratory. It is astonishing to think that prior to Koch there was no agreed system for testing and proving the hypothesis that a particular organism caused a disease. He devised a system of rules that had to be satisfied before that conclusion could be drawn. These were, and still are, known as the Koch–Henle postulates. Koch said that to prove that an agent caused a disease, you needed to be able to find the organism in every case of the disease. Then you needed to be able to culture the organism in vitro, in the laboratory. Next, you had to infect, usually by injection, another victim with the cultured organism, and cause the disease. Finally, you had to retrieve the organism from your artificially infected victim.

Now that doctors had several new means of determining the cause of many infections, death certificates marked as 'The Bloody Flux' began to seem impossibly flaky. With scientific discovery came scientific rigour, both in diagnosis and record-keeping. However, if it were simply a matter of a change of name, from 'Flux' to 'dysentery', then the disappearance of the diagnosis would be an irrelevance. People would still have been dying from the illness. So why did fatal diarrhoeal diseases start to vanish?

The first, simple answer is public health. The widely held view is that public health originated with the anaesthetist John Snow's observations on cholera in London's Soho. However, our supposedly primitive ancestors arranged their lives in complex and sophisticated ways to protect themselves from infection. Lavatories dating from about 2800 BC have been found on the Orkney Islands; others from about the same date have been excavated in India, in Pakistan and in the Palace of Knossos, on Crete. There are areas of the world where such public health arrangements are yet to be matched. The Cloaca Maxima, Rome's great drainage system, was begun in the sixth century BC. In AD 70, during the rule of the emperor Vespasian, marble public urinals were erected in Rome with a small charge for entry. Public lavatories in London were not constructed until 1851, for the Great Exhibition; the Ladies' were in Bedford Street and the Gents' in Fleet Street. In Rome, by AD 315, public lavatories were well established. These were social as well as functional, places where people conducted business and discoursed. Ten to twenty people could be seated around a room, with their wastes being washed away by flowing water.

Toilet paper was being used in China as early as AD 589. Clay water pipes first came into use in Pakistan, in the Indus Valley, around 2700 BC. The Egyptians were using metal water pipes in around 2450 BC; the Palace of Knossos had clay pipes constructed around 2000 BC. The Romans acquired their first aqueduct in 312 BC. At their height, there were ten aqueducts supplying 250 million gallons of water each day; per capita about twice what a citizen in a modern European city might use. Much of the water was directed into fountains and public baths. The senate appointed a water commissioner, who was responsible for seeing that the water supply was kept adequate and clean; the punishment for contamination of the water supply was death. Following the Great Fire of AD 64 – the one through which Nero is meant to have 'fiddled' – Rome was rebuilt with broad streets and open public squares that were easily cleaned by officials called the aediles. They also imposed strict regulations to control the sale of rancid and unfit foods.

Nonetheless, the Romans had no more clues about the true cause of infectious disease – whether by water, food, insects or airborne – than their pre-Victorian counterparts almost 2,000 years later. If the water supply in the aqueducts became infected, they were completely unprotected. Pre-Christian Roman disease protection and treatment largely comprised prayer to a huge panoply of specific deities, one for each disease. As has been stated in the introduction, many lives were prematurely curtailed by infectious disease. Indeed, the fall of the Roman Empire may have been hastened by successive epidemics, possibly bubonic plague or smallpox. Even more tragically, many millions still die prematurely from infectious disease, many of them children. Some estimates quote figures of 15 million preventable child deaths from infectious diseases per year. Many of these deaths would be preventable by means known to the Romans – indeed known to mankind, for almost 5,000 years.

What was it like to have the Bloody Flux? There is a recorded account in the Bible, in Acts 28:8, where the father of Publius lay ill with fever and bloody diarrhoea. He was cured by the laying-on of hands. It seems unnecessary to detail the symptoms of diarrhoea, but the feature of dysentery is fresh red blood in the stools. As in the case of Publius' father, there may be fever, together with abdominal pain and weight loss. Without treatment, the symptoms may be prolonged and fatal; abscesses may appear in the liver or indeed elsewhere in the body. In a gruesome culinary metaphor, the pus from such abscesses is said to resemble anchovy paste.

The Bloody Flux – and infectious diarrhoea in general – vanished from the West as a major cause of death for a number of reasons. The most important was improved hygiene, in the form of sewer systems, which channelled effluent away from water supplies. We should contrast the experiences of different parts of London in the nineteenth century to illustrate this point. In 1853–4 the city suffered a devastating attack of cholera. Over 10,000 died. It was to be some years before the cholera bacterium was identified, and even this was not the impetus behind the great engineering works undertaken by Joseph Bazalgette, chief engineer of London's Metropolitan Board of Works. That incentive was the distaste of Members of Parliament for the foul stench emerging from the neighbouring Thames in the Great Stink of 1858. By 1866, the majority of London was served by proper drainage into treatment works, instead of the previous rank channels that simply emptied into the river. The scheme did not extend to London's East End, and in that year there was a cholera epidemic in that region alone. This is what modern scientists would recognise as a case-control study, if an unethical one; afterwards, the theory that cholera was carried in foul water – Snow's original hypothesis – was generally accepted. There was a further epidemic in Hamburg in 1892. London was spared, and Bazalgette was credited with saving many thousands of lives. Between 1848 and 1872, 10 deaths per 1,000 in England and Wales were registered with the Government Register Office as being due to 'cholera' (without microbiological confirmation this probably included other diarrhoeal diseases). By 1901, there were no such recorded deaths.

Hygiene has been improved in other ways that have contributed to the disappearance of the scourge of death by diarrhoea. For example, human faeces is no longer used as an agricultural fertiliser. In most western nations, food suppliers are inspected for the quality and storage of their merchandise, much like the supervisory role of the Roman aediles. Should you suffer real Bloody Flux in the form of amoebic dysentery – and it still occurs throughout the West, including about 500 cases per year in New York State alone – then it may be treated. Simple replacement of lost fluid may be life-saving, although to cure the illness antibiotics may be necessary, especially if spread occurs to the liver where those anchovy-paste abscesses may form. Infectious diarrhoea remains a very common disease, but rarely kills where there is access to medical care. The troops of Napoleon's Army as they marched on Moscow were not so lucky: the ultimate failure of that campaign owed as much to diarrhoeal disease as it did to military defeat and the weather. *Entamoeba hystolytica*, the cause of amoebic dysentery, remains the third leading parasitic cause of death in developing nations.

Other diseases in addition to the Bloody Flux have also mostly vanished from the western world. Some, such as tetanus, have relatively simple explanations. Nowhere is this better illustrated than in dreadful outbreaks of tetanus following the tsunamis of Boxing Day, 2004. Tetanus is a terrifying disease. Once symptoms develop, it is almost uniformly fatal. The bacterium, *Clostridium tetani*, produces a potent toxin that paralyses the muscles of movement. Death is by asphyxia, as the muscles that move the lungs become incapacitated. The word 'tetanus' is derived from the Greek *tetanus*, meaning a muscular spasm, from the verb root *teino*, meaning to stretch.

Tiny injuries, invisible to the naked eye, may harbour a fatal inoculum of tetanus bacteria. The portal of entry may not be visible in 20 to 30 per cent of cases. A classical case often taught to medical students is of the elderly lady who develops peculiar neurological signs some time after pruning her roses; a tiny thorn splinter is enough to introduce the lethal invader. Deadly poison leaks out that prevents vital chemical signals being passed along nerve endings, paralysing muscles. Tetanus also has the folk-name 'lockjaw', because the muscles of the face and neck are often affected, giving rise to a terrifying fixed smile – the so-called 'risor sardonicus'. If the patient can be kept alive for long enough for these delicate nerve fibres to recover, survival may occasionally be possible.

Clostridium tetani, like most of the *Clostridium* bacteria, favours the airless world immediately below the surface of soil. It is often shed in the stools of livestock and humans. Immunity to tetanus can be acquired in two ways, one more reliable than the other. Vaccination, as most people know, is routinely performed in most developed countries. The vaccine was developed by the Frenchman Descombey in 1924. It was rapidly taken up and used to enormous benefit to prevent the disease in wounded soldiers, many of whom would have had soil-contaminated injuries, during the Second World War. The efficacy of the toxoid is demonstrated by the incidence of tetanus in soldiers when compared to the war of 1914–18. During the earlier, pre-vaccination conflict, there were 13.4 cases per 100,000 injuries. By 1939–45, the figure had fallen to 0.44 per 100,000. The pre-vaccination death rate may be estimated by the mortality in the developing world, which may be as high as 28 per 100,000. In North America, the figure is less than 0.1 per 100,000. The first dose of vaccine is usually given in childhood, with boosters in later life. The other means of acquiring immunity is through regular exposure to the soil, perhaps through tilling and husbandry. Although effective, the latter is a less reliable means and unvaccinated farmers will still be at risk. Nonetheless, immunity does increase with age, although waning in later life, as in the case of our rose-growing elderly lady. Thus, in the catastrophic floods of the 2004 tsunami, where many were injured both seriously and trivially by floating debris in sewage-contaminated water, it was the children who were particularly at risk.

In Thailand, where there is an effective and modern healthcare system, most children were vaccinated against tetanus and there were no tetanus cases. In Indonesia, however, where healthcare is primitive and haphazard, there were many susceptible children. Nobody knows for certain how many died of tetanus in the whole region following the Boxing Day tsunamis, but it seems certain that the figure was in the hundreds. Without the sophisticated intensive care equipment required to maintain the respiration of affected individuals, it was almost always fatal.

This disparity perfectly illustrates how this particular Quiet Killer has been all but totally vanquished in countries like Britain and the United States. Tetanus is utterly preventable by immunisation with the toxoid. This toxoid is extremely cheap and very easy to produce – all that is required is treatment of the poison with formaldehyde. Changing social patterns, with fewer people involved in farming and soil work, would inevitably have changed the pattern of disease spread. This may not have been entirely beneficial as fewer people exposed to the soil would mean more susceptible, and there would still be many deaths following inevitable trivial, everyday injuries. The few cases that do still occur in developed countries tend to be in adults aged over 50 in whom immunisation was inadequate or never performed, or occasionally in heroin addicts. Nonetheless, to the shame of the world, up to half a million deaths from tetanus still occur in the developing world each year. Newborn children who acquire infection from the umbilical stump account for 70 to 80 per cent of these.

There are similarities here with diphtheria. This is a singularly unpleasant condition. It is really an infection of the throat and nose, although disease may arise in the skin. The word derives from the Greek for leathery hide, and refers to a characteristic grey-white membrane which forms over the site of infection, usually the palate. Hippocrates described the condition in the fourth century BC. The Greek physician Aretseus describes diphtheria thus: 'The tonsils are covered with a white, livid, or black concrete product.' He noted that diphtheria may cause massive damage in the throat, which can be so severe as to cause death by strangulation; death may occur on the first day if the trachea (windpipe) is affected. However, as in tetanus the bacterium *Corynebacterium diphtheriae* var. *gravis* produces a poison, which is lethal to the heart, nerves and kidneys. Unlike tetanus, however, diphtheria only seems to prey upon man, and is not found elsewhere in nature. Death is usually by poisoning of the heart. A particularly cruel feature of the disease is the tendency for children to die suddenly, up to eight weeks from the initial symptoms, when they had apparently recovered from the throat infection. Nowadays, diphtheria is treatable even when the infection is established; a combination of antibiotics and the antidote to the poison may, although not always, be life-saving. The antitoxin was first used in London in 1891, and when used on a wider scale the mortality promptly fell from 63 per cent in 1894 to 12 per cent in 1910. The discovery of the antitoxin is credited to Emil von Behring, a German physician who had worked with Koch and Ehrlich. The toxin of diphtheria had been extracted from cultures of the organism. It was von Behring's brilliant deduction that an anti-toxin might be generated by injecting sub-lethal doses into animals. The consequent toxin–antitoxin combination proved safe and life-saving; further to this, uninfected individuals might, after injection, develop immunity and never again suffer the disease. Von Behring won the first ever Nobel Prize for Medicine for his work.

In affluent countries, this frequently fatal disease of childhood has declined dramatically in the years following the Second World War. In 1920, in the United States, there were 152 cases per 100,000 population. By 1980, this had fallen to 0.002 per 100,000. Improving social conditions – better housing, ventilation, hygiene and so forth – have indubitably contributed to the decline of diphtheria. The predominant route of spread is through the air, in infected droplets of water breathed out by a victim or a carrier. Epidemics have been transmitted through milk, but this is rare. When people become more affluent, when slums are cleared, and when fewer children and families need to share rooms, then such airborne infections do tend to wane. Certainly the incidence of diphtheria began to fall prior to the introduction of an immunisation programme. However, there is no doubt that the vaccination has massively accelerated the decline of the condition, and changed its nature. In highly immunised populations infection occurs more commonly through the skin, through minor injuries, more like tetanus. Outbreaks have rarely occurred in such populations, suggesting that the decline in the disease has many causes. Sadly, once again, in a pattern which must be becoming familiar to the reader, the disease remains common in some parts of the world. There was an unexpected surge of cases from the countries of the old Soviet Union, as the once rigid bureaucracy of communism faltered.

Readers will by now also be developing familiarity with a weary litany of diseases that are treatable or preventable by simple measures, yet persist in the developing world. This will be dealt with more fully in Chapter Three. However, the world may, provisionally, pat itself on the back over the extinction of one major killer from the past. Smallpox, a scourge that probably killed more children in Europe in the late seventeenth and early eighteenth century than any other illness except the 'Flux', was finally eradicated by massive global effort in 1979, the last cases being in Bangladesh, Ethiopia and Somalia.

What was it like to have true smallpox in its *major* form? (See Chapter Five.) Classical accounts described five forms: haemorrhagic, flat, ordinary, modified and *Variola sine eruptione*. The characteristics were a feverish illness with chills and backache about two weeks after exposure that lasted through the illness. In the ordinary form there was subsequently a pustular rash, much like chickenpox, except the blisters were deeper. Where there was a rash it would tend to last about two weeks (if death did not intervene) and the skin would be shed with scars left in its place; these could be disfiguring. Bleeding could occur into the pustules. Death was inevitable in this malignant haemorrhagic variant, the black pox. In the flat form death would intervene before rash developed. In modified smallpox (varioloid) and *Variola sine eruptione* a mild version of disease would develop in patients on whom vaccination had been performed. A fictional account, from the meticulously researched novel *The Speckled Monster: A Historical Tale of*

Battling Smallpox by Jennifer Lee Carrell, gives as accurate an account of confluent smallpox as any: 'Eleven days in, Lady Montagu entered the critical stage of confluent smallpox. In places, strips of skin peeled away; elsewhere, boils erupted as secondary infections attacked the raw, stagnating wounds. A brown crust crept over her whole body; from under the scabs leaked pus stained rust with blood. What little was left of her skin felt sheeted in flame as her temperature jagged higher . . .' (p. 52). Fatal smallpox could arise from overwhelming infection with the virus itself, from bleeding, or from other complications such as pneumonia or asphyxia from obstruction of the inflamed larynx.

Historically, smallpox seems to have appeared in Europe in around the sixth century and, catastrophically, in the Americas in the sixteenth. Here again is an example of a Quiet Killer altering the course of history. Cortés was able to subjugate the hugely numerically superior and militarily competent Aztec nation in Mexico once the scourge had almost annihilated the indigenous population. There were cases in China, India and Africa at far earlier dates, from at least 3000 BC. The mummy of Ramses V is said to bear scars of the disease. It was a major cause of death in the West until effective vaccination was introduced in the seventeenth and eighteenth centuries, an advance which almost certainly contributed to dramatic population growth.

The virus now persists only in laboratory conditions in the Center for Disease Control in Atlanta, Georgia, and in Russia; as far as is known, these are secure. There have been reports that some specimens may have fallen into less responsible hands. This will be discussed more fully in Chapter Five.

The presence of the smallpox virus in laboratory conditions led to one of the oddest and most tragic episodes in the history of that terrible virus. The world's last ever smallpox outbreak occurred, in 1978, not in Karachi or Johannesburg or Yangon, but in Birmingham, as a result of the accidental release of such artificially stored stocks. It is a story of intellectual vanity, of terrible coincidence, and of hubris and honour that would not be out of place in Greek melodrama.

The department of medical microbiology at Birmingham University was then chaired by Professor Henry Bedson, son of another famous microbiologist, Sir Samuel Bedson. Henry had been anxious for his laboratory to be accredited as a Smallpox Collaborating Centre, with all the kudos that would entail. The world, however, was changing. The World Health Organization knew that the end was in sight for its eradication programme. It wanted to limit the number of laboratories that were handling smallpox, especially old-fashioned laboratories where security and containment facilities for hazardous pathogens were dated; the sole safety precaution in such aged facilities was vaccination. Bedson's application had been rejected. He still wished to continue and complete his smallpox research programme, which he thought important. But he knew his time was short. Safety facilities had certainly been improved since his early days, when the deadly virus had been handled on open benches. He decided to step up the pace of his research before the inevitable closure of his laboratory following a WHO inspection.

The floor immediately above the lab where smallpox was handled was occupied by the Department of Anatomy. A service duct ran from the Virology lab to the Anatomy Department's telephone room. Smallpox had occurred in the Anatomy Department before: a medical photographer from the Department had contracted the disease in 1966. That episode had been carefully investigated, and it was concluded that the victim had probably been infected through his varied social contacts. At that time, smallpox was still occasionally being imported into Britain – there had been an outbreak from Karachi as recently as 1962.

Janet Parker was a medical photographer from the Department of Anatomy at the University of Birmingham. On Tuesday 15 August 1978, she developed a skin rash. This was not the beginning of her illness; her first symptoms had begun the previous Friday, with muscle pains and headache. Over the following days, she began to feel more and more unwell; her rash progressed despite the antibiotics her GP gave her. By 24 August, she was so unwell that she was taken to hospital. Fluid was taken from the blistering rash that was by now more or less covering her body; smallpox was confirmed. She was transferred to the local smallpox hospital, but died a little less than two weeks later. Her mother, with whom she had stayed during her illness, was admitted to the same hospital on 7 September with smallpox, despite having been vaccinated on 24 August.

An investigation into the outbreak was announced. Before this could happen, before Janet Parker's death, and before the admission to hospital of Janet Parker's mother, Henry Bedson took his own life.

Why was smallpox extinguished, while other infectious diseases persist? There are others that you might have thought would be more readily wiped from the face of the earth. TB, for example, is usually curable if properly managed, whereas there is no known effective treatment for smallpox. Measles is, like smallpox, a viral disease, preventable by vaccination, which still kills in both developed and developing countries. So what was so special about smallpox?

The name Edward Jenner, the father of modern vaccination, is inevitably key in the history of vaccination and smallpox. The story is so well known as to be almost folklore. On 14 May 1796, in his surgery in Berkeley, Gloucestershire he inoculated two three-quarter-inch scratches in the forearm of a boy, James Phipps, with fluid from the pock of a milkmaid, Sarah Nelmes, who had cowpox. The boy suffered a mild illness seven to nine days later, but remained well. On 1 July, Jenner deliberately infected the boy with smallpox. He still remained completely well.

Jenner was not, in fact, the first to deliberately vaccinate with cowpox. In the graveyard of the beautiful church of Worth Matravers, Dorset lie the remains of Benjamin Jesty. Little of the fabric of Worth Matravers has changed over the years, and you can still read Jesty's incredible story laconically recorded upon his gravestone. Jesty was a farmer. In the spring of 1774, there was a terrible outbreak of smallpox in his parish. Jesty was desperate to protect his pregnant wife, Elizabeth, and his two sons, Robert and Benjamin. The Jestys had two dairymaids on their farm, both of whom had previously had cowpox. During the mild illness that followed, these girls had to nurse family members through the smallpox epidemic. Neither, noticed Jesty, fell ill with smallpox. Jesty surmised that if accidental cowpox protected from smallpox, then so would deliberate infection. He decided to give it a go.

Jesty collected 'matter' (pus) from the udder of a cowpox-infected cow and with the point of a darning-needle he scratched the pus into his wife's arm. He repeated the procedure with his two boys. All were spared smallpox. Furthermore, the boys were re-inoculated with smallpox fifteen years later, and suffered no ill effects. It is almost certain that Jenner knew of Jesty's experiment; in the 1770s, he was working in the south-west of England, although not in Dorset.

Jenner's genius lay not in making the intellectual leap between infection with cowpox and protection from smallpox, but in his patient, thorough methodology. He wanted, in the best traditions of his profession, to be sure at first that he would not injure his subjects. In the twenty-year period between learning of Jesty's bold, but uncontrolled and potentially dangerous, feat and inoculating the boy Phipps, Jenner carefully investigated the effects of cowpox infection. Following the success of his early experiment, he decided to repeat it in a series of subjects. He was delayed by the unfortunate temporary absence of cowpox from Gloucestershire, but by 1798 he had data from twenty-three successfully vaccinated subjects and decided to publish his findings under the title 'An Inquiry into the Causes and Effects of the Variolae Vaccinae, Discovered in some of the western Counties of England, particularly Gloucestershire, and known by the name of Cow Pox'.

Despite the clear benefits of vaccination, there was controversy over the procedure from the outset. There was opposition from those with a vested interest in the competing method of variolation, where individuals were inoculated with pus from patients with mild smallpox (known by its Brazilian name, alastrim). This was a practice which had been carried out, in, for example, China, since at least 1000 BC. The church fulminated against the immorality of introducing an animal disease into man. Others raised the possibility of accidentally introducing other animal diseases into humans. Nonetheless, even though not all the population was vaccinated, the procedure was notably successful. Even in an epidemic year, mortality from smallpox fell to 148 per 100,000 from a pre-vaccination peak of 400–500 per 100,000.

The World Health Organization was formed on 7 April 1948. It immediately decided to address a number of problems including smallpox, and embarked on a massive worldwide search-and-destroy vaccination programme. Apart from that laboratory accident in Britain in the 1970s, the campaign was massively successful. The very last naturally acquired case of smallpox occurred in a hospital cook in Merca, Somalia. His name was Ali Maow Maalin. He had, by chance, been a vaccinator in one of the World Health Organization eradication teams. His rash struck on 27 October 1977. He was lucky: he survived. Smallpox acquired in the wild in endemic areas tended to have a mortality in the order of 20 per cent. Following a safety period of surveillance, on 8 May 1980 Resolution WHA33.3 was signed at the eighth plenary meeting of the 33rd World Health Assembly. It declared that the world and all its people were free from smallpox. Occasional reports of sporadic cases of smallpox in Central African countries have transpired to be monkeypox, a superficially similar and indeed related condition.

Why has eradication not been possible with the other Quiet Killers? Smallpox had several features that made it ideal for an eradicative vaccination programme. First, it has generally been believed that immunity is lifelong and a second infection is not possible. This is not strictly true, but re-infection was rare enough to mean that epidemics could not ensue in highly vaccinated populations. Next, true smallpox is an acute illness with obvious visible symptoms and signs, where there are few long-term silent but infectious carriers. Chronic illnesses such as TB, where people may be infected and infectious for years without obvious symptoms, are massively harder to eradicate. The fact that smallpox had a high mortality – about 20 to 30 per cent – meant that there was generally high public support for vaccination, although in many countries this had to be supported by compulsory legislation. Smallpox vaccination was mandatory in Britain until 1948. Crucially smallpox, in its virulent form, has no known animal reservoir.

41

Yet the strangest feature of smallpox eradication remains the sheer serendipity of the vaccine. As I have said, Jenner's story is so well known as to be practically folklore. Like most folklore, however, it is mostly wrong. Smallpox was probably not eradicated by cowpox, but accidentally, by modified smallpox virus, and through the unconscious agency of a man Jenner himself regarded with loathing.

Dr William Woodville worked in the London Smallpox and Inoculation Hospital. Cowpox inoculum was scarce, and it was noted that it tended to lose efficacy when passed from person to person. Resistance to the idea of direct inoculation from animals meant that vaccination was performed arm to arm, one patient's pock being inoculated into the arm of the next. Only the first in this chain would have been directly infected from the cow. Variolation had been carried out by this system for years, it having been noted that the system of 'removes' further modified the virulence of the infection. When, in 1799, Woodville discovered cowpox among two cows at a local dairy, he acted quickly and vaccinated seven locals with 'matter' from these animals. He then inoculated them with smallpox – but crucially, and the source of Jenner's loathing, after only five days. Jenner would always wait at least a month before testing his vaccination with smallpox.

Woodville discovered that some of the many hundred subsequent vaccinees were more ill than he expected. One child even died. Jenner believed that from Woodville's sloppy practice, cowpox had become contaminated with virulent smallpox. Whereas nowadays there would have been public outcry and a press scandal, the mortality from smallpox was so desperate in 1799 that Woodville suffered no opprobrium save that of Jenner.

If the smallpox vaccine that was subsequently used by the WHO to eradicate the disease is examined by sophisticated gene-sequencing methods, it may be seen that it more closely resembles smallpox virus than it does cowpox. Something happened to the vaccine virus at some point to make it genetically closer to the disease it was aimed to extinguish. That potentially dangerous accident would almost certainly have made it more effective as a means of inducing immunity. Probably by trial and error, subsequent vaccinators arrived at a safe version of this modified virus.

The vaccine that the WHO used for global eradication derived from stock originally acquired by Professor Benjamin Waterhouse in Boston, Massachussets in 1800. He was sent the strain from a Dr Haygarth of the vaccination hospital in Bath, Somerset. From whom did Haygarth obtain his virus? Dr William Woodville, of the London Smallpox and Inoculation Hospital. What did Jenner think had happened to Woodville's virus? It had become contaminated by virulent smallpox.

It is impossible to know if the chain of events I have described is completely accurate, although it is biologically and historically plausible. One thing is clear, though. This series of coincidences could not occur in our age. Jenner's original experiments would have been rejected out of hand by any modern ethics committee, without whose approval no human research can progress. Vaccinees would not have been deliberately re-challenged with smallpox, allowing the possibility of mixture of wild smallpox and vaccine in the same person. Even if this happened, the chances are that it would be impossible to transfer the hybrid virus to another individual. Arm-to-arm vaccination, with its consequent passage through living subjects, would be illegal; this was banned in 1881, as it was realised that diseases such as erysipelas, impetigo, TB and syphilis could be transmitted in this way. We now know that even more dangerous infections like hepatitis B and HIV may be similarly transmitted. The vaccines would nowadays be tested and re-tested at every stage to ensure they were pure; any suggestion of contamination of a vaccine with a living and dangerous virus would cause a scandal. Such a situation has already arisen with commercial rabies vaccine. Smallpox vaccination is not completely safe; indeed, following an imported outbreak in Britain in 1962 almost as many died from complications of vaccination as died from smallpox. Jenner's vaccine would not be licensed in the twenty-first century. We could not today repeat the process by which the most successful vaccine of all time was developed.

Of course, we might not need to. Plenty of highly effective modern vaccines have been developed using our more advanced modern knowledge. As will be discussed later, the best hope for a vaccine for the threatened epidemic of 'bird flu' lies in reverse genetic engineering. This is a complex concept which I shall explain fully in Chapter Seven. Such technology was beyond the wildest imaginings of Jenner and Woodville. It has to be remembered, though, that these sophisticated techniques have not yet yielded vaccines for other ancient killers such as TB, nor for newer ones like HIV. And the fact remains that one of the greatest of the Quiet Killers was vanquished by a combination of diligence; international cooperation; the unlikely genius of a farmer; incompetence; luck; and finally, trial and error.

The greatest of these is luck. Compare smallpox with measles, for instance. Measles is, potentially, a killer. It has a mortality of about 1 in 1,000 cases in the developed world; deaths may be from pneumonia, acute measles encephalitis or from a singularly unpleasant condition called Subacute Sclerosing Panencephalitis. This causes inexorable mental decline and inevitable death some years after the infection. Can it be prevented by vaccination? Good luck: yes. Is there, as in smallpox, a measles-type virus that just happens to cause harmless disease in humans, which could be easily used for vaccination? Bad luck: no. (Although measles virus is closely related to canine distemper virus.) In fact, real measles virus is used for vaccination, only specially attenuated to be harmless. So why isn't measles a candidate for eradication, like smallpox?

The real reason that measles is not a candidate for worldwide eradication is that it is just not a serious enough problem for the wealthy. We think of measles, despite its risk of death, as a minor childhood illness. We forget that, both historically and currently, measles is a major killer. There are several reasons for this, which shed further light on the subtle, stealthy, opportunist nature of the Quiet Killers. The first is that measles, like many other infections, is far more severe in the malnourished. The mortality of 1 in 1,000 may be amplified many times where people are poorly fed and have little access to clean water and fresh produce. Poor nutrition leads to depression of the immune response. From being an inconvenience, an illness characterised by rash, runny nose and a few days of misery, measles becomes a lethal harbinger of pneumonia, blindness, gangrene and deafness. Severe mouth ulcers may worsen the malnutrition, as feeding becomes impossible. Where there is deficiency of Vitamin A, the cornea – the clear part of the eye – becomes weakened; measles may cause it to rupture.

Measles is less of a killer in developed countries, paradoxically, because it used to be more common. A feature of infectious diseases is that they do not behave identically among all populations. Malaria, to be discussed later, may cause a fairly mild disease among people who are constantly being reinfected; recurrent exposure leads to protective, if temporary and somewhat unreliable, immunity. Conversely, an unprotected, previously unexposed westerner visiting a malarial area may develop a fatal infection at the first bite. Infectious disease physicians will tell you that it is sometimes difficult to convince visitors from tropical countries to take malaria prevention when they leave for their native lands – this used to be known as 'British Council' malaria, because cultural visitors to Britain would often fall ill when they returned home as their immunity waned. Exposure over many generations may even favour genetic adaptations to malaria. Sickle cell disease, for instance, protects from infection with the parasite.

With measles, in many countries the reverse is the case. In the West the disease has been present for many generations. During that long period virus and victim settled into a state of 'balanced equilibrium'. The majority of the population would have some form of immunity. This would be acquired either from previous, true infection or from immunity transmitted from mother to child. This sort of maternal transmission of immunity is generally considered to be transient. However, it may well mitigate the worst effects of the disease, especially if the infection occurs early in life. This means that measles is less severe in areas of high endemicity. Not so in other countries, though. Measles behaves quite differently in populations where it is not endemic.

Where it had never previously been encountered, the consequences were disastrous. The Aztec Empire was at its height in 1519 when Hernán Cortés landed at Veracruz. The population then stood at 5 million. By 1521, it had fallen by a third. The vast majority of the deaths occurred not by military action, or massacre, or even malnutrition, but by disease. Ultimately there were believed to be 50 million deaths among native South Americans from infectious diseases following the arrival of the Spanish. Foremost among these diseases were smallpox and measles. We will find out in later chapters – particularly in Chapter Seven – more about why the Quiet Killers behave differently in populations who have never before encountered them. However, the pattern was repeated throughout populations where the white man brought his viruses – the Pacific and Australasia were decimated.

Every few years, however, in countries with endemic measles, enough people would be born who had no long-lasting immunity to provide sufficient susceptible individuals to permit an epidemic. Without vaccination, this would lead to cyclical epidemics of mostly mild disease every five years or so. Thus the disease and immunity of the population – the so-called 'herd' immunity – were in near balance. The period between epidemics would tend to define the age at which most victims were infected. So if an epidemic were to occur every fifty years, then most generations would be affected. However, a cycle of five years, as with measles in Europe, would mean that infection would tend to occur mainly in children. These children would probably have some residual maternal immunity and would therefore have mild disease. A paradoxical effect of imperfect vaccination is that the epidemic cycle tends to lengthen; thus the age of infection tends to increase. This may have serious consequences. Some infections like chickenpox are more serious in adulthood. Rubella, another viral disease, generally causes a harmless illness with rash. However, it can lead to severe birth defects if acquired when pregnant. A poorly controlled rubella vaccination programme in Greece led, in 1993, to that country's worst ever outbreak of congenital rubella. Carelessly controlled vaccination had simply raised the age at which young women tended to catch the disease, and more of them were then likely to be pregnant.

When diseases do 'vanish', like civilisations, the end is often very rapid. A disease may even be eradicated if some people remain susceptible. Smallpox was eradicated without 100 per cent coverage, not by mass vaccination but by an obsessional search for outbreaks and individual cases and their containment by isolation and targeted vaccination. The mathematics of this is complex, but it relies on a phenomenon called the Transmission number, or R0. The R0 basically refers to the number of cases that may be infected from each primary case. If the number falls to less than one, then an epidemic will peter out. There are a number of ways of reducing the R0. One is not really feasible in humans – a ring cull of infected and susceptible individuals: basically, you kill all the known victims as well as potential victims before they are infected. Such a method was used to control the 2001 foot-and-mouth epidemic in Britain. Next is isolation of all infected cases. Ring vaccination will have the same effect as ring culling, as long as the vaccine is sufficiently reliable. Where treatment is available, that reduces the duration of infectivity, which will in turn reduce R0. There is no treatment that will reliably treat smallpox. Many believe that the antiviral agents cidofovir and ribavirin may work; as yet no case has been treated, because the disease was eradicated before the drugs were invented.

There is one other Quiet Killer which may be heading the way of the dinosaur and the dodo. Polio, the paralysing virus which put President Franklin Roosevelt in a wheelchair, is targeted for global eradication within the foreseeable future. Like many of our Quiet Killers, this is a disease with a long history, with representations of the characteristic withered limbs appearing in ancient Egyptian hieroglyphics. Yet it was not described in western medicine as a distinct disease until the eighteenth century – perhaps surprisingly, as it is one of the few once-common diseases to cause sudden paralysis among children. The condition was not identified as being infectious until 1908, when Landsteiner and Popper identified the virus. It was to be almost fifty years before an effective vaccine was produced, during which time there were numerous epidemics within western nations, particularly among servicemen stationed in unsanitary conditions during the Second World War. The virus is transmitted in faeces. The story of polio vaccine development is littered with false starts and disasters, where the disease itself was introduced accidentally in some cases. By the late 1950s, there were two effective vaccines available: the injectable variety, a killed vaccine developed by Jonas Salk, and the oral vaccine, designed by Albert Sabin, which is a live but damaged virus. There were 58,000 new cases of polio in the United States in 1952. By 1964, after a widespread vaccination campaign notably backed by Elvis Presley, the figure had fallen to 121.

The Director-General of the World Health Organization from 2003 to May 2006, South Korean Lee Jong-wook, announced in March 2003 that the wild polio virus could be eradicated from the human population within three years. He based his prediction on the dwindling number of recorded paralytic polio cases, and the fact that 99 per cent of the cases occurred in a single country – India. That country then had a faltering mass vaccination campaign and the WHO believed that kick-starting it, and improving the vaccine coverage in other countries such as Egypt and Pakistan, might lead to its eradication. Like smallpox, polio has no animal reservoir. The WHO has, however, estimated that some 10,000 laboratories worldwide carry stocks of the virus; these will have to be destroyed, just like Henry Bedson's smallpox virus. There is also the small risk that Sabin's oral polio virus vaccine can revert to its dangerous, wild type in 1 in every 2.5 million cases. The injectable Salk vaccine does not have this complication. However, it is more expensive and tends to have a lower uptake.

There is a snag to Lee Jong-wook's prediction. In October 2003, the governors of three states in northern Nigeria – Kano, Kaduna and Zamfara – decided to suspend polio immunisation until the vaccines were investigated and proven safe. The motive behind this suspension was not the proven small risk of the Sabin vaccine reverting to its dangerous state, but something far more nebulous and troubling. Many Muslims in the north were so indoctrinated by a number of fanatical imams that they believed that polio vaccination was being used as a ploy by western countries to inject people with noxious chemicals to reduce their fertility or infect them with HIV or AIDS. Polio has undergone something of a local resurgence as a consequence. The WHO reported that more than 40 per cent of the 677 new cases of polio recorded worldwide in 2003 were in Nigeria. Identical strains of the polio virus have appeared in several neighbouring western and central African countries, including Benin, Togo, Ghana, Burkina Faso, Cameroon and the Central African Republic. In 2001, polio had reached an all-time low, with only 483 cases reported worldwide. By August 2004 alone, there were 1,004 cases, almost all in predominantly Muslim countries or their immediate neighbours.

Polio has another continuing legacy. Even in the United States there are estimated to be 600,000 people living with the long-term consequences of polio infection, including muscle withering, paralysis, fatigue, chronic pain and cold intolerance. The worldwide figure is probably in the order of ten million.

Leprosy has vanished from most western nations, and not for entirely explicable reasons. Also known as Hansen's disease, it was the first ever disease to have a bacterium definitively associated as a cause and was once endemic in Britain and Europe. It may be argued that leprosy does not belong among the Quiet Killers; many believe that it is deforming but rarely fatal. This is not so – people with the lepromatous variety of leprosy have a mortality of four times that of the general population. King Henry IV of England is said to have died of leprosy.

Why leprosy disappeared from Europe is not clear, but then the means of transmission of the disease is not clear either. It is certainly associated with poverty, rural residence and not wearing shoes. Occasional cases arise in North America through contact with the nine-banded armadillo. Leprosy disappeared in many countries coincident with industrialisation; the current WHO eradication programme relies on seeking cases and treatment with combinations of antibiotics. This is a disease with a fair chance of eradication.

There is another method by which a Quiet Killer has all but vanished, and that method is poorly understood. Rheumatic fever was once among the great terrors for parents of young children. It has waned in recent years, although the bacterium which causes it has far from disappeared. It is a strange condition, where the body becomes a victim of friendly fire. Substances in the coat of the causative agent – *Streptococcus pyogenes*, also known as Group A *Streptococcus* – so resemble our own tissues that there is overlap in the response of our immune systems to the infection. Our white cells cease to recognise some of our own body parts as our own and start to attack them. In rheumatic fever it is the heart that is irreversibly damaged. However, something has happened to *Streptococcus pyogenes*. It is still a dangerous bacterium, causing severe skin infections and the so-called 'flesh-eating bug' necrotising fasciitis. But it seems to have more or less abandoned causing rheumatic fever. Nobody really knows why this should be. Bacteria do mutate among populations to alter their virulence, both upgrading and downgrading. Outbreaks do occur now and again. There have been a few cases in American military training establishments. Some think the drop in virulence is due to widespread prescription of antibiotics, but nobody really knows for certain. Our Quiet Killers may move in mysterious ways.

And dropsy? This is an old-fashioned term for heart failure. Heart disease is diminishing as a cause of death in many western nations. Some doctors even believe that it is caused by one of the Quiet Killers. This will be discussed in more detail in Chapter Ten. But dropsy as a diagnosis has gone the same way as the Bloody Flux. That's not to say you can't die of it; but you've got to die of something.

Following our relatively upbeat beginning, we will now move on to more depressing territory: the Quiet Killers that are coming back or changing their distribution.

TWO

Rabid Returners
Diseases that are coming back or changing their distribution

The world is changing, and at a more rapid pace than ever before. Whether or not you believe in the doctrine of global warming – and it becomes ever harder not to – the world is changing in other ways too. Humans are migrating across the planet in their millions, driven by the search for prosperity. The speed of travel is almost miraculous by historical standards, and the numbers travelling by air are huge. It is said that up to a million people may be airborne at any single time. This is reflected in figures for imported 'exotic' diseases into western countries. In 1971, 1,010 cases of malaria were imported into countries around the European Union. By 1997, that number had risen to 12,328. Sexual behaviour has changed too: for better or for worse, the age of first intercourse has diminished in most nations and the number of sexual partners over a lifetime has increased. All of this means that the ecology of disease has changed and will continue to change. We have looked at diseases that have, for whatever reason, gone away. It is now time to look at those which may be coming back or threatening new areas of the world.

Many think that changing climate patterns will mean that diseases once endemic will come to haunt us in the West again. In Britain, we already get about 2,000 cases of malaria per year, almost all imported. There are rare cases of 'airport malaria', where a baggage handler or unlucky passer-by is infected by a rogue mosquito that has hitched a ride from some infected spot of the globe. The Quiet Killers may be even more capricious, random and bizarre in their mode of transmission. There has been at least one outbreak among patients in a hospital in Britain, from where malaria was eradicated in the 1950s. In 1999, three patients contracted *falciparum* malaria in a Nottingham hospital; one died. None had visited a malarial area. It transpired that the source was almost certainly a contaminated vial of saline – a junior doctor had drawn up the solution to flush some drips and used the same bag for four people. The first patient had the disease and inadvertently passed it on to the others.

Malaria has appeared in literature since the earliest times, being mentioned by Aristotle, Chaucer, Shakespeare, Defoe, Pepys, Homer, and many others. There are descriptions of malaria-like symptoms in Chinese writings of 2700 BC. These descriptions have common themes in keeping with the diagnosis: intermittent fevers alternating with shaking chills, lassitude, enlarged spleens, pale skins. Such are the markers of the disease; we will return to its mortality. The historical consequences of malaria have been dramatic. We have mentioned Cromwell. St Augustine, first Archbishop of Canterbury, probably died of malaria, as did Dante and at least two popes. Military campaigns have collapsed due to malaria. There were said to be 1.2 million cases in the American Civil War alone.

While the diagnosis from the ancient scribes mentioned seems likely, it is only in relatively recent times that the parasite was identified. For generations, the cause of the disease was a mystery. Tsar Peter the Great of Russia attempted to control malaria in his soldiers by banning the eating of melons. The Frenchman Laveran is widely accredited with the discovery of the parasite, in 1880. The British military physician Ronald Ross won the 1902 Nobel Prize for identifying the mosquito as vector at the end of the nineteenth century, although the Italian Grassi and the great tropical physician Manson deserve at least as much glory.

During the 1850s, between 12 and 60 per 1,000 admissions to London's St Thomas's Hospital were due to malaria. That is a far cry from the total sum of 2,000 imported cases per year that we are now seeing. There are four species of malaria that afflict humans: *Plasmodium falciparum*, *P. vivax*, *P. ovale* and *P. malariae*. The first two are by far the most common, and *falciparum* is known as malignant because it is the greatest killer. Could malignant malaria again afflict western nations?

We should pause for a moment to examine why malaria disappeared from most of the western hemisphere, because that will give insight into whether it will come back again. There are species of mosquito which are capable of transmitting malaria in most western nations. But they don't. Why not?

The life cycle of malaria is complex. It has several phases in its transmission, reproducing and maturing both in the mosquito and in the victim. It requires more than just a susceptible person. One victim is simply not enough – effectively to persist in a population, a pool of infected people is required. If that pool falls to low enough numbers, malaria transmission collapses. Precisely this happened in Britain and Europe during the 1880s. The weather was actually passing through a warmer phase in this period; the decline in transmission cannot thus be attributed to climate change. Malaria had in fact been endemic in Europe during the so-called 'Little Ice Age'; this is reflected in references to the disease in writers of the period including Shakespeare, Pepys and Defoe. Malaria probably disappeared for reasons to do with human behaviour. Land drainage disrupted mosquito breeding sites. Mechanisation of farming reduced the numbers of labourers on the land, limiting the exposure of humans to infected mosquitoes. Farmers developed new techniques of maintaining cattle through the winter by feeding them root crops, such as turnips and mangelwurzels, which store well. Not only did this mean that less time would be spent harvesting and thus exposing oneself to mosquitoes, but it also made it likely that those same insects would bite uninfected cattle instead. This was a period of rapid advance in building technology. Better buildings protected from mosquitoes. The use of quinine became more widespread as a treatment as it fell in price; effective treatment kills the parasite in the blood and reduces transmission.

Malaria was declared eradicated from Europe in 1975. The last case in England was in the 1950s. Eastern Europe lagged behind the wealthier western nations in this respect. It required DDT, the first modern pesticide, to eradicate malaria from Finland, Poland and

Russia after the Second World War. Malaria was probably introduced to the United States by European colonists and African slaves in the sixteenth and seventeenth centuries. The move of the capital from Jamestown to Willamsburg was probably prompted by malaria. It became endemic in many areas of the country as the continent was colonised. In 1934, 125,556 cases were reported. The decline in malaria before the introduction of extensive vector control measures was probably much the same as in Britain. In 1947, a malaria control programme was introduced which, by using indoor spraying with DDT, was able to effectively eradicate malaria from the United States, where it was still endemic in thirty-six states including Washington, Oregon, Idaho, Montana, North Dakota, Minnesota, Wisconsin, Iowa, Illinois, Michigan, Indiana, Ohio, New York, Pennsylvania and New Jersey. You may be certain that after such efforts unexplained episodes of malaria in western nations would elicit a vigorous and effective response from such public health bodies as the Centers for Disease Control.

At present, then, the risk of malaria becoming re-established in the western hemisphere is remote. The only European states that contain malaria are south-western Turkey, Turkmenistan and Armenia. The nearest with the more lethal *falciparum* variety is Tajikistan. Malaria was once nearly eradicated from these areas; the reasons it is back are more political than climatic. The collapse of the old Soviet Union has meant that control programmes have folded. In Turkey, hydro-electric schemes have meant that there are wide expanses of standing water which act as breeding grounds for the mosquito vector. While it would be hasty to categorically state that malaria will never come back, it seems unlikely. There are over 400 species of *Anopheles* mosquitoes. Only about seventy of these transmit malaria. The species of mosquito required to transmit lethal falciparum do not, at present, dwell in most developed nations. Of the malaria-carrying species, only *An. atroparvus* occurs in any numbers in Northern Europe, with *An. freeborni* and *An. quadrimaculatus* occurring in North America. The most efficient malarial vector *An. gambiae* (efficient because it prefers humans to cattle) is largely confined to sub-Saharan Africa. Even should suitable mosquitoes migrate, the malaria parasite requires stringent climatic requirements to reproduce. *Falciparum* malaria requires a temperature of 24°C for 11 days for the vital part of its life cycle called sporogony reliably to complete in the mosquito (it may occur less reliably at lower temperatures, but this is the optimum; below 18°C it cannot occur). This would require a pessimistic prediction for global warming. You could compare the likely return of malaria to the cooking of a soufflé. While a hot oven is necessary for your soufflé to rise, the careful preparation of the ingredients is just as vital.

Malaria really belongs in the category of diseases that have never gone away in the undeveloped world, or that of diseases that have vanished in the West, although sporadic unexplained cases do occur in some countries, including the United States. Troublingly, there is convincing evidence of malaria resurgence in Africa, particularly Kenya, Rwanda and Tanzania, and at increasing altitudes in the South American Andes. The reasons for this are complex. Other factors may be involved, for instance civil unrest, human migration and the reluctance of many countries to use DDT. Many firmly believe though that rising global temperatures are causative. Further, according to WHO other insect-borne diseases like Dengue are spreading north parallel with climate change.

Are there any illnesses which might genuinely be coming back? TB is famously resurgent in the West, with recent outbreaks in London and New York. Cynical observers have commented that this resurgence is barely a novelty in many parts of the world where between 2 and 3 million deaths occur annually, and that it has simply been that infection among middle-class white citizens of western countries has concentrated the mind of western governments. It is certainly true that the notifications for TB have been steadily rising in London, for instance, since 1995. Some of this represents a rump of people – the homeless and the indigent – in whom we may never eradicate the disease. However, there is more to the story than this, and it will be considered more fully in the next chapter. The real concern about TB is not that it is coming back, but that is is becoming untreatable.

Syphilis, chlamydia, genital herpes and gonorrhoea are increasing explosively in incidence in the western world as sexual mores change. The incidence of all four doubled in England, Wales and Northern Ireland from 1995 to 2000. In the United States, the figures are less clear; some estimates put the incidence at 15 million new cases per year, an increase of 3 million since 1996. The figures are similar in other European countries. Sexually transmitted infections peaked immediately after the Second World War, then receded for the period 1950–60. Since then, there has been a progressive rise with a more recent dramatic increase. Almost certainly all official figures are an underestimate. Many sexually transmitted infections have no symptoms, and thus do not present for treatment. They also kill only rarely, although gonorrhoea may have a fatal septicaemic variety and syphilis untreated will eventually kill in a proportion of cases.

I do not propose to discuss the signs and symptoms of any of these treatable venereal diseases because they are not killers. There are those that are: HIV and human papillomavirus, the cause of cervical cancer. They are discussed elsewhere. However, I will briefly discuss syphilis, a disease that once ravaged the world and is certainly returning, with a 1,058 per cent increase in the UK between 1995 and 2003. Not for nothing was it once known as the Great Pox, to distinguish it from the smallpox. There is a description of the disease in Voltaire's *Candide*: '[A]s Candide was walking out, he met a beggar all covered with scabs, his eyes sunk in his head, the end of his nose eaten off, his mouth drawn on one side, his teeth as black as a cloak, snuffling and coughing most violently, and every time he attempted to spit out dropped a tooth.' Syphilis is a bacterial disease that may lay dormant for many years, but eventually may cause inflammation in just about any part of the body. The commoner sites of disease were the brain and spinal cord, causing profound mental disturbance and damage to the nerves, as well as to the great blood vessels around the heart. Syphilis appeared explosively in Europe in the fifteenth century, but from exactly where remains uncertain. Some say it was a New World import; others that it was a common illness that suddenly upgraded its virulence. Two facts about syphilis are clear, though: it was widespread and it caused great suffering. In the United States, the peak incidence was during the Second World War, for reasons that may be obvious, when in 1945 there were over 500,000 cases, or about 72 per 100,000. Deaths from untreated syphilis, with inexorable mental decline, must have been horrible to observe. Syphilis altered the conception of disease among doctors forever. From the outset, it was recognised that the illness arose from outside the body and was a 'thing' in its own right. This completely challenged the previous notion of disease being caused by derangement in the balance of the 'humours'. While it was to be hundreds of years before the bacterium was identified, and even longer before an effective cure was discovered, this understanding paved the way for a new approach to disease causation closer to that which we recognise today. It was also the impetus for the setting-up of many hospitals for the incurable, some of which survive in altered form in European cities today.

No disease was as convincingly disarmed by Fleming's penicillin as syphilis. By the 1950s, it had become a curable disease and the incidence had plummeted. But now, syphilis is most definitely coming back. The incidence in the United States has risen from its trough of 4 per 100,000 in 1950 to approaching 20 per 100,000 today. In Britain, between 1999 and 2002 there were 481 confirmed cases of syphilis in Greater Manchester, a massive increase over previous years. This was extensively investigated, and a number of disturbing features emerged. Put briefly, the main reason the outbreak happened was that gay men were having frequent, risky and unprotected casual sex. I met one of the authors of an official report into the episode. He told me that while unravelling the course of transmission of the disease they attempted to document the source of patients' likely contact with syphilis. They did so by identifying known locations for casual sex encounters – gay saunas, for instance – and counting up the number of sexual partners each patient had at each site. My colleague told me that some of the patients had difficulty in providing detailed information for the study. Some men had no idea how many casual sexual partners they might have had over a given period as they were so numerous; double figures over a weekend were not uncommon. Of the gay men who were diagnosed with syphilis, 37 per cent were HIV-positive. Syphilis is readily transmitted by oral sex; in this study, only 7 per cent of respondents used a condom during that act.

It is clear that attitudes have changed towards risk-taking behaviour in sexual activity among gay men. This has been corroborated by surveys throughout the developed world. The availability of effective treatments – if not actual cures – for HIV seems to have had an unexpected payback. During my time in HIV medicine, I heard the view expressed in certain quarters that you were not properly 'gay' unless you were HIV-positive. There are websites given over to the practice of 'bare-backing', which means deliberately having unprotected sex with someone you know to be HIV-positive in the expectation of catching the virus. As a physician, I find this point of view challenging to say the least. Of course, it would be inaccurate to attribute the enormous increase in sexually transmitted diseases observed in many western countries to gay men. Increased incidence has similarly been observed through heterosexual activity. One of my duties as a microbiology doctor was to contact the GPs of patients newly diagnosed with chlamydia, syphilis, herpes or gonorrhoea. It became depressingly routine to observe the dates of birth of some of these patients, many of whom were contracting STDs in their early teen years. At that age I was still climbing trees. This is not a moral judgement. However, from my point of view as a physician, aware of the possibility of long-term consequences of STDs such as infertility and ectopic pregnancy, these telephone calls made for a sorry chore. It was also sometimes my task to inform and support people newly diagnosed with HIV. It was both depressing and shocking to me that people should still be acquiring the virus despite the widespread publicity and public education that are designed to prevent it.

HIV is tragically changing its distribution at the gates of western Europe – in eastern Europe there are estimated to be in excess of 1.2 million infected. The decimation of sub-Saharan Africa by the virus is barely news. More than 20 million people have already died of HIV infection, with probably more than 60 million infected. Five million new infections occur every year, 800,000 of these in children. Worldwide, over 70 per cent of infections are acquired heterosexually and 10 per cent by intravenous drug use, the latter particularly in countries such as Spain and Portugal which failed to introduce needle exchange schemes early. Such schemes were introduced in England and Wales in 1987. The prevalence of HIV here is in the order of 1 per cent of drug-users, even among the higher-risk prison population. Portugal did not begin such harm reduction strategies systematically for almost fifteen years after this date; the prevalence among its prisoners is estimated to be 11 per cent.

The increase in incidence in non-HIV sexually transmitted diseases is worrying because some of the consequences of infection are equally dangerous. Human papillomavirus – the agent of warts – is, as we have said, incontrovertibly linked with cervical cancer. This is particularly of note because there is now an effective vaccine available. An estimated 471,000 new cases of cervical cancer are diagnosed each year worldwide, with 80 per cent of these occurring in the developing world. Screening has reduced the incidence in developed nations; nevertheless, there are nearly 3,000 cases of this preventable condition in the United Kingdom each year.

Probably the ultimate current example of a disease which is changing its distribution is West Nile Virus. Many infectious disease physicians are on tenterhooks to be the first to diagnose the condition in Britain, and it does seem that it is only a matter of time. West Nile Virus is not a new disease. Indeed, as I mentioned in the introduction, some have suggested that Alexander the Great may have died from it. It was first described in Uganda in 1937. The harbinger of its arrival in the West was the symbolic bird of prophecy, the crow. Illness in humans around New York City Zoo was linked to multiple deaths of that bird. Subsequent surveillance relied in part on testing dead crows for the illness. In a bizarre misprint at the time, one newspaper reported that it was not crows but cows that were dying and tumbling from the trees. In fact, all corvid birds may be infected, including jays, ravens and rooks.

West Nile Virus is a dangerous disease. It may be harboured by other mammals, including horses. Pigs and dogs may be infected without symptoms, but infected pregnant ewes abort. The vector is the mosquito, and unlike the related flavivirus of Yellow Fever this virus is not especially choosy about which mosquito it hitches a lift with. The widespread genus *Culex* may carry it; culicine mosquitoes occur throughout the world with the exception of the northernmost temperate regions. *Culex* also transmits filariasis (the agent of elephantiasis) and Japanese encephalitis (discussed in Chapter Ten). The significance of its ubiquity is that once a West Nile Virus infected pool is established, the ultimate spread across geographical space is almost inevitable. Furthermore, other species, including mosquitoes tolerant of colder climates like *Coquillettidia perturbans*, may also carry the virus. So it has been no surprise that the United States has been serially infected county by county like falling dominoes. Cases have also occurred in Canada. The first cases were recorded in New York in 1999. By 2004, more than forty states had been affected. In 2002, there were more than 4,000 victims of West Nile Virus in North America. This is the largest outbreak ever recorded. The states with the highest numbers of confirmed human cases were Illinois, Michigan, Ohio, Louisiana and Indiana. In 2005, there were 2,949 cases; about a half had simple fever and another half had full-blown brain inflammation (encephalitis). There were 116 deaths.

It might be tempting to blame the development of infections previously unseen in geographical areas on climate change. Such is not the case with West Nile Virus. In this condition we have susceptible populations, a suitable vector and introduction of the new virus. That is all that is required; in this respect, viruses are different to more complex parasites like malaria or sleeping sickness. Nobody knows exactly how West Nile Virus arrived in North America, but the initial disease cluster around the zoo has suggested importation from an exotic species. However, this has never been proven.

In case you are reading in Europe and imagine yourself safe, think again. West Nile Virus has occurred in much of southern Europe. Cases have occurred in Italy, with cycles of disease in the summer. There was an outbreak affecting seven humans and five horses in the Camargue, in southern France, in October 2003. This region is peculiarly susceptible to the disease because of a combination of estuarine mosquito habitat, migratory wildfowl, proximity to North Africa and numerous both wild and domestic horses. West Nile Virus appears to be migrating northwards.

Anxiety about West Nile Virus, although understandable, has tended to overshadow other similar emerging mosquito-borne illnesses. Eastern equine encephalitis is, as its name suggests, harboured by horses but may cause brain inflammation in humans along the eastern states of the Union. It has a mortality of 35 per cent, and a third of those who survive are left with lasting neurological damage. There are also St Louis encephalitis, western equine encephalitis, Venezuelan equine encephalitis, and several others. These are spread by biting insects, with a variety of animals as reservoirs including bats. I sometimes think it is better not to know too much about these diseases because too much information may cause you to lock your doors and never venture out into the dangerous world inhabited by sick animals and mosquitoes again. The symptoms are broadly similar: feverish, self-limiting flu-like illness in some with a proportion progressing to encephalitis as headache, confusion and even death. I would make two important points before you panic and lock yourself away. The first is that these diseases remain rare. The second is that the apparently high mortality and incidence of long-term consequences conceals a bias. The simple fact is that milder disease tends to pass below the statistical radar. Many people with mild fever and headache do not consult a doctor at all. Most people with encephalitis are taken to the doctor by a friend or relative. This means that the infections are probably more common and milder than is suggested by the figures; indeed, when blood donors were screened after the Camargue West Nile Virus outbreak, a small number of people with undiagnosed disease was discovered.

The opposite is true of one of my favourite Quiet Killers, rabies. Once rabies has caused symptoms it is almost invariably, and horribly, fatal. Infections are therefore not common or mild. We have discussed rabies in the introduction, on the basis of its ability to alter human behaviour across enormous disparity of scale in order to ensure its transmission. Rabies has been a subject of medical literature for millennia. The ancient physician Celsus identified saliva as the source of transmission during the second century AD. He used the word 'virus' in this connection for the first time. The WHO estimates that 10 million people per year are treated after exposure to rabies. Some 40,000 to 70,000 people are thought to die of the disease each year, many in India. There is a major current resurgence in China, where it has overtaken TB and AIDS as a cause of death. Rabies transmitted by vampire bats continues to be a serious problem in the cattle industry in South and Central America and vampire bat bites continue to be a cause of human rabies infection in rural areas. Is the disease coming back or changing its distribution?

The rabies vaccine has been available since Pasteur developed it 150 years ago. Rabies was eradicated in many parts of Europe and North America before the Second World War by vaccination of dogs and the rounding-up of strays. There are two reasons why the situation is now possibly reversing. First, the virus has adapted to the fox as a reservoir and today just about any mammal may become infected with rabies. The second wildcard in the pack is the bat. Lyssavirus – almost identical to rabies, with similar mortality – has been found in bats in Britain. There was a death in Dundee in 2002 of a man who handled bats.

Several islands have been traditionally free of the virus: the United Kingdom, New Zealand, Australia, Japan and Hawaii. There are five to six human cases per year in the United States, usually transmitted from bats, although thousands of infected wild animals such as raccoons, skunks, coyotes and foxes are found each year. Rarely, a case arises through transplant of contaminated tissue. There was a disastrous example of this in Germany recently, where at least three people were infected with rabies from an infected donor who probably caught the illness in India.

Could rabies re-establish itself in Britain? The last cases of animal rabies in Britain – excluding two Daubenton's bats, in 1996 and 2002, and a dog that contracted the disease in quarantine – occurred in animals imported into the United Kingdom by soldiers following the First World War. There is a modern programme to eradicate or at least control the disease in foxes in Europe, based on spreading bait laced with oral vaccine. However, that programme has only been partly effective. In March 2005, there was an increase in rabid foxes in Germany and France because the programme was only patchily enforced. Already in Britain about 2 per cent of Daubenton's bats in Scotland have antibodies to European bat lyssavirus. The theoretical concern is that an infected fox could introduce the disease having walked through the Channel Tunnel, or that a wild or domestic animal or even a human could become infected by eating or handling an infected bat.

So, yes, rabies has shown a slightly worrying trend, but at present the risk is relatively small. However, there is a further scientific reason for fearing the disease. Almost certainly, the disease originated in bats and mutated to infect other animals. Rabies is an RNA virus. Because such viruses lack proofreading mechanisms, they are among the fastest-evolving organisms. They thus produce diverse viral populations, ready to explore new hosts or escape defence mechanisms. For this reason, RNA viruses cause two of the six leading infectious killers, namely AIDS and measles, and are implicated in two others, acute respiratory infections and diarrhoeal diseases. Of the forty-two emerging or re-emerging infectious diseases between 1996 and 2000, twenty-three (55 per cent) were caused by RNA viruses.

The rabies threat remains theoretical and small. So if I, as an infectious diseases physician, had to choose a specific potentially resurgent Quiet Killer, which would it be? My answer may surprise you. There is quite a list to choose from. Avian flu is probably the biggest potential threat in terms of the numbers that could be affected; this is dealt with in more detail in Chapter Seven. HIV of course has cut a catastrophic swathe through sub-Saharan Africa, and continues to sweep almost unchecked through eastern Europe and Asia. West Nile Virus has now affected every state of North America; it is marching relentlessly across Europe and will undoubtedly reach Britain in the near future. Bacteria resistant to almost every antibiotic are becoming increasingly common, both in hospitals and the community; the prevalence of resistance among one of mankind's greatest enemies, TB, climbs ever higher. 'New' killer infections such as Nipah virus and Hendra virus, discussed in Chapter Ten, present us with alarming new challenges.

Yet my answer to the question posed above, though, would be . . . measles. You may think this an odd choice. Most of us think of measles as an almost trivial illness; an inconvenience. Even the name itself sounds benign, almost a nickname. But there are several reasons for taking this viral condition far more seriously. We have already seen that measles caused catastrophic mortality among populations of the South Pacific and Australia when first the infected white man came among the unexposed natives of those lands. But those days have surely gone?

Actually, they haven't; measles is the world's foremost cause of vaccine-preventable deaths. The most accurate available figures put it at number 6 in the world league table of mortality by cause – immediately below TB and malaria. Children in the developing world are dying from the virus at the rate of 800,000 per year. Measles even continues to kill in the western world. There was an outbreak in Dublin in 2000. Although more were probably affected, 355 cases were proven by laboratory testing. Of these, 111 needed admission to hospital. Thirteen were so sick that they required the intervention of an intensive care unit. Seven needed to be artificially ventilated – a tube placed down the throat so they could breathe. Three have died, so far. But measles is a cruel disease; as you will find out, this may not be the end of its story.

Measles is highly infectious. We have already encountered the figure called the R0, or transmission number. This is the number of people likely to be infected from the first infected case. Measles has an R0 value of between 11 and 14. This is a higher figure than for either influenza or smallpox, both of which are considered highly infectious. This means that where there is a collection of unvaccinated people, of whatever age, then there is a very high chance that they will develop the disease.

As we have said, measles is a virus. It belongs to a group called the morbilliviruses, and as such is related to Hendra virus, Nipah virus and canine distemper virus. It is spread in droplets of breath and it replicates in the lining of the airways. From there, it is transported by white blood cells to every part of the body, including the skin and brain. The symptoms are fever and rash. There may also be cough, sore eyes and runny nose. Children with measles are often absolutely miserable. Sometimes there are characteristic spots inside the cheeks. You might have thought that the condition was easy to diagnose, but one study has shown that 50 per cent of all measles diagnoses made by family doctors turned out to be wrong.

Most previously healthy people with measles recover and are then immune for life. However, a number of potentially lethal complications may develop. Measles causes a paradoxical reaction within the immune system. On the one hand, the white cells produce an effective and rapid response that clears the infection and provides long-term immunity. On the other hand, it knocks the immunity for six, and for a very long time. Protection from other infections, especially pneumonia, is crippled. Antibiotics and vitamin A may help, but not always. This was the reason why our unfortunate Dubliners needed the intensive care unit, and why three of them died. It does not take a mathematician to calculate the proportional mortality: 3 out of 355, or slightly less than 1 per cent.

Measles also infects the brain. There may be three consequences from infection at that site. Acute inflammation, or encephalitis, at the time of the initial infection may be fatal (in 15 per cent of cases), or may cause long-term brain damage (in 20–40 per cent). A small group of unlucky patients who had measles in the past may, coincidentally and unrelated to the viral infection, go on to develop leukaemias. These people are prone to developing a condition called measles inclusion body encephalitis. This causes prolonged fits; 85 per cent die and 15 per cent are left with long-term epilepsy or other complications. Finally, and most viciously, six to eight years after the measles infection a condition called subacute sclerosing panencephalitis (SSPE) may develop. This causes inexorable mental deterioration, fits and inevitable death. There are very few 'always' in doctoring, but I will stick my neck out and say with certainty that everyone with SSPE will die.

So why am I so concerned about measles? These complications are (relatively) rare. Another infectious, vaccine-preventable condition, bacterial meningitis, has a higher mortality of up to 5 per cent, even with treatment. Measles encephalitis affects 1 in 1,000; SSPE 1 in 1 million. Shouldn't I save my anxiety for more commonly lethal conditions?

Let us dwell for a moment on the causes of the 2000 Dublin outbreak. We know that measles will tend to occur when vaccination coverage falls below a certain threshold percentage. To completely eradicate transmission, uptake of 95 per cent is required. In Dublin, the coverage had fallen to 79 per cent by 2000. Although at the time of writing the situation had slightly reversed, uptake of the recommended measles vaccine programme has been dropping in Britain consistently since 1998. It had fallen to 84 per cent (although this trend may be reversing slightly); in some areas, it has been as low as 60 per cent. Recently the 'Cochrane' evidence on the combined measles–mumps–rubella (MMR) vaccine has been published. There is, currently, no higher authority of evidence in Britain that can be produced in support of a medical treatment. That study has shown that doubts about the safety of the MMR vaccine are unfounded. The extraordinary part of this is that they had to do so, as though the whole medical profession were somehow divided on this issue. They are not. Doctors overwhelmingly agree that MMR is safe, and with plenty of sound evidence to do so. Meanwhile, new diagnoses of measles in Britain have trebled. There is a hobby horse available here; I shall not mount it except to recap some figures from the experience in the United States. That nation suffered a measles outbreak in 1989–91, as a consequence of poor vaccine coverage. The result was illness in 55,622 people, mostly children under five years, requiring more than 11,000 hospitalisations and killing 125 sufferers. Here is why I am so concerned: for the first time, despite repeated reassurances to the contrary; despite convincing scientific evidence confirming the safety of the vaccine programme; despite serious criticisms of the probity of the source of the rumours, some sections of the public have decided that they know better, and that they do not need to follow the advice of 'experts'.

Mumps has also emerged recently, among university students in Britain. There has been some suggestion that this has been connected with falling MMR uptake thanks to the scare over autism. This is not so; most students entering university would not have been given MMR, which was introduced in 1979. Mumps is not a wholly benign condition, either. Some of the students suffered an unpleasant encephalitis. Both pancreatitis (a potentially lethal inflammation of the pancreas, where the body practically digests itself) and inflammation of the testicles (causing sterility) may occur, although the latter is relatively rare.

Measles bucks the trend of emerging infectious diseases in not being transmitted by animals. About three-quarters of the illnesses under surveillance by the Center for Emerging Infectious Diseases are zoonoses. Many are covered elsewhere in this book.

You will have gathered from the tenor of this chapter that I consider the impact of global climate change a minor player in the development or spread of infectious disease and that our anxieties about their resurgence are overwhelmed by the existing killers. What seems to me far more important is unified political will in tackling the common killers. A single death from a rabies-like virus in Dundee, although tragic, is firmly put in perspective by the global mortality from malaria and diarrhoeal disease. We will discuss some of these diseases in the next chapter.

THREE

Here to Stay
Diseases that never went away

The great influenza pandemic of 1918 killed more people than the First World War. There have been many epidemics since, and influenza has never gone away. Why do these great epidemics happen? Why are we so worried about bird and pig flu? As for malaria and TB, were we just complacent when we thought they had gone away, when millions still died every year in the developing world?

There is no shortage of Quiet Killers that continue to stalk us. I am conscious of a certain repetition when I say that there is a clear difference between the developed and the developing world in this respect. Some diseases have been vanquished in the richer countries but continue to wreak havoc in the less fortunate nations. Leprosy is a good example. Unfortunately, as we have observed, nobody is absolutely certain why leprosy has vanished from many, usually richer, parts of the world. One could make a very long list of all the Quiet Killers that still stalk the world; the indexes of most infectious diseases textbooks are many pages long. Of course, many of these are very rare; some have not been seen for many years. However, it is only smallpox that we can say with any certainty has vanished. I will use this chapter to discuss examples of diseases that are still problematic throughout the world, to emphasise the reasons.

The Quiet Killers that have the greatest impact throughout the world are infectious diarrhoea, malaria, HIV and TB. Why can these illnesses not be controlled in the same way that smallpox was, and polio may yet be?

The answer, in a word, is vaccines. Smallpox vaccine was developed by near accident in a way that simply would be

impossible today. The methods that Jenner used would be unaccept-
able to modern ethical committees, without whose approval no
research on humans may progress. That is not to say that scientists
are not hunting for vaccines for these conditions. There are, though,
major scientific difficulties with deriving such vaccines for them. We
will examine each in turn and discuss why they are hard to control
and why it is that this Holy Grail is so elusive. I will also discuss
other vaccine-preventable conditions as illustration of principles
relevant to vaccination.

The impact of diarrhoeal diseases, past and present, is huge. They
have significantly affected the course of history through their effect
on military campaigns. The Crusades of the eleventh and thirteenth
centuries frequently almost failed due principally to diarrhoea and
typhus; in wars up to the American Civil War of 1861–5, deaths
from diarrhoeal diseases tended to exceed those from military action
by at least two to one. Diarrhoeal diseases have an enormous list of
possible causes, some vaccine-preventable and some not. For
example, a new vaccine for rotavirus, a very common and sometimes
fatal cause of diarrhoea, is currently being considered for all
American children. Of course, in the developing world access to
clean drinking water and available, cheap rehydration for people
with diarrhoea would potentially save millions. The American Civil
War was the last major campaign to be fought before the germ
theory of disease was widely accepted. Of note, though, was the
observation that 'miasmas' and 'effluvia' (diarrhoea) were believed
to be implicated in transmission, and efforts to protect troops from
such contamination actually meant that the two-to-one ratio of
disease versus wounds as a cause of death was much lower than in
previous wars. Lord Lister began to publish his experiments with
carbolic disinfection in 1867, and the understanding that humankind
needed to be protected from its own sewage was becoming well
established. Nevertheless, diarrhoeal disease remains a major hazard
in war and peace. The Gallipoli Landings failed as least as much due
to the incapacitation of soldiers with diarrhoea as to military
incompetence. It is a measure of the fact that the 'Flux' has such a
variety of causes that even in modern campaigns with assiduous

hygiene, such as the recent Gulf War, diarrhoea remains trouble-some. During the disastrous French campaign in Indo-China, which preceded the Vietnam War, there were 160,000 cases of amoebic colitis (the Bloody Flux) as well as numerous cases of diarrhoea due to salmonella, shigella and cholera. While it may be possible to offer cholera vaccination in an endemic area, developing catch-all vaccines for other causes is limited by the variety of agents of disease.

TB is a paradoxical disease because it is simultaneously advancing, retreating and staying the same, even in the same countries. The research which led to my PhD concerned TB and stress. I recall two major responses when I told people what I intended to study. My parents, who were at university in the 1950s, were told that they would never see a case of human TB. The other absolutely standard reply was, 'TB. That's on the way back, isn't it?' I have discussed elsewhere TB as a disease that is coming back or changing its distribution. Here, I shall discuss it as a disease that has never gone away, because it illustrates a number of points about the Quiet Killers and how they wax and wane.

TB is, usually, a chronic disease; that is, one of long duration. With a few exceptions – pneumonia and meningitis when caused by the tubercle bacillus, for instance – the illness is protracted and slow. TB may also become dormant. In fact, in 90 per cent of cases this is precisely what happens. Infection usually occurs in childhood. The resulting illness resembles the common cold and may even pass unnoticed. The bacillus is then able, like Rip van Winkle, to sleep for decades. Many people die at advanced ages of unrelated disease, totally unaware that they ever had the infection. In 10 per cent of people, however, the infection may reactivate. When it does so, it may be in a huge variety of forms and just about any organ of the body may be infected. If the illness reactivates in the lungs, it is infectious, although the most transmissible form infects the larynx. In the two years it takes someone with untreated pulmonary TB to die, they will transmit the bacillus to ten other people. This is one of the key reasons why TB has never gone away, and probably never will do. There is an amazing statistic to be included here: 50 per cent of the world's population is infected with TB. You can imagine, then, that with 10 per cent of those reactivating every year then eradication is a challenge, to say the least.

And yet we came so close. In the period after the First World War to the end of the twentieth century, notifications of TB in western countries plummeted. The reasons for this – improved sanitation, effective treatment – are discussed elsewhere. However, there is a further reason why TB waned in the west, and is rising elsewhere. That explanation owes more to mathematics than to biology.

Let us now compare two hypothetical infectious diseases. One arises abruptly, acutely and causes a short-lived illness which kills only a proportion of its victims. It is highly infectious: all previously unexposed people will contract the disease. Protective immunity follows an attack. We do not need to name the illness, but measles would do as well as any. Without intervention, such an illness will cause epidemics every few years, as a new population is born that has no immunity. The regular interval between each epidemic is known as its 'periodicity'. In the case of a highly transmissible, acute illness that affects principally children, the gap between epidemics will be short. The periodicity of measles is about four years. Our second illness is chronic, of low infectivity and progresses slowly. This disease will tend to have much longer gaps between the peaks of the epidemic, because protective immunity will develop far more slowly in a community. Diseases such as TB have a periodicity that may be measured in centuries rather than years or decades. This effect is exaggerated because TB transmission shows a peculiarity: schoolchildren between the ages of about 5 and 13 are relatively protected from the disease. This is the so-called 'safe school age'. Schoolchildren are excellent amplifiers of disease, as they collect together in large numbers in close contact. Armies may serve the same function; indeed, the 1918 Great Influenza Pandemic was massively amplified by returning demobilised soldiers.

Why should schoolchildren be protected from TB? I shall digress for a moment to explain. We know that TB is highly influenced by the hormones concerned with stress. Our white blood cells are partly at the mercy of stress hormones; the chemical most closely involved with chronic stress called cortisol affects these cells almost as though it makes them drunk. Coincidentally, alcohol itself has similar effects when taken in excess. Alcoholics are especially susceptible to TB. We know that TB tends to reactivate during conditions of stress; at time of war, for example. Like most biological systems, the stress response has a naturally occurring antidote. The action of cortisol is partly antagonised by a chemical called dehydroepiandrosterone, or DHEA. This chemical fluctuates naturally during life. It is present in low concentrations from birth to the age of 5, then increases as the adrenal gland matures. It is present in high concentrations until puberty, when much of it is converted into sex hormones. DHEA then wanes again after the age of about 50. This is the age at which dormant TB tends to reactivate; many think these two phenomena are related. The largest reservoir of active TB in most western countries is not, as many believe, immigrants, although they have certainly increased both the incidence of disease and the proportion with resistant TB. It is the indigenous over-50 population whose immunity is faltering because of their falling DHEA production. Some scientists believe that DHEA represents something close to the elixir of eternal youth. Indeed, in one laboratory, technicians took to spooning it into their tea. The only discernible consequence was that the males became balder. I should caution against such experiments, especially as DHEA is freely available on the internet. Nobody knows for certain what the consequence of excess DHEA might be on your cells; some people believe it may predispose to certain kinds of cancer. DHEA also diminishes in advanced HIV disease. This may be part of the reason why patients with AIDS suffer from TB many times more frequently than HIV-uninfected people.

The periodicity of TB is responsible for some of the paradoxes concerning the wax and wane of the illness. TB was declining in Europe and the West before the advent of improved sanitation, treatment and vaccination. It is probable that we were on a declining curve of the epidemic and that was accelerated by social changes and technology. Other parts of the world are at a different stage of the epidemic cycle. Somalia, for example, is either on the ascending curve or near the peak. This was so marked that at one hospital where I worked it was facetiously suggested having the phrase 'you have TB' printed in Somali for the benefit of all patients presenting with an unexplained feverish illness from that country. Ireland may be slightly behind the rest of Europe in passing the peak of the current epidemic, which may explain the traditionally higher prevalence of the disease there. Of course there are political, historic and cultural reasons why the Irish may have had more TB than the English and Welsh. There are also genetic elements. Some scientists have calculated that 90 per cent of susceptibility to TB is genetically determined. But the natural fluctuation of disease in populations is a crucial element in its spread; for once, we should not wholly blame ourselves in the developed world for the geographical variation in prevalence of a Quiet Killer. Whether westerners introduced TB to some parts of the world is another matter.

There is another reason why TB might be a disease that has not gone away, even in the West. There has always been a small rump of the destitute, homeless and dispossessed whom even advanced socialised care will fail. Even during the absolute trough of the cycle of TB in Britain, about 2,500 cases per year were notified to the public health authorities. This is certainly an underestimate; 50 per cent of cases of fatal TB in Britain are not diagnosed until post mortem. Both London and New York have recently been rudely awakened by epidemics of TB in their midst. Much of this is imported, and worryingly some of it is resistant to the drugs. However, there is little doubt that the dismantling of supposedly redundant social schemes for the control of TB in New York contributed to the problem in America. Some cynically suggest that the problem was only taken seriously when a few white, middle-class citizens were affected.

It may come as a surprise to some to learn that there is no effective vaccine against TB. Readers in many countries may bear a scar, usually on the upper arm, from the BCG vaccination. BCG stands for Bacille Calmette–Guérin, and is a deliberately damaged or attenuated strain of a bacterium related to TB called *Mycobacterium bovis*. In theory, it works by providing a not-quite-TB stimulus to the immune system. Why does this not qualify? Was the painful injection with its frequent attendant discharge and pus simply a waste of time? Some countries – the United States, for example – do not use it at all. The question of whether or not it works has been the subject of much debate. Large international studies pointed to a paradox. It seemed to work in some countries, but not in others. In Myanmar (previously Burma), for example, it seemed to make people more susceptible to TB, not less. In Britain, it is believed to confer some temporary protection but is particularly effective in preventing the highly dangerous variety that causes meningitis. The current thinking is that our immunity is 'primed' by contact with TB-like bacteria which live in the environment. This is discussed further in Chapter Six. It means, though, that BCG is a far from perfect vaccine.

We should take a moment to explore the nature of vaccines and the nature of TB to see why creating a vaccine for this illness is so difficult. Vaccines work by preparing the immune system for a specific infection. In doing so, obviously, they evade the need to actually suffer the disease. Once a naturally occurring infection has been introduced to the body, our white cells – specifically, the lymphocytes – retain a prolonged memory of the encounter. Once the imprint is stamped into the cells' design, it allows a far more rapid immune response should the infection attempt to recur. The cells do so by processing markers on the surface of the infecting organism. If we can decipher exactly which markers encourage these 'memory' cells to store their imprinted blueprint, we can purify them and simply use harmless fragments of the Quiet Killer to produce the same immunological response as would result from a real infection. In practice, the development of vaccines has often been more primitive than this would suggest, as simply damaging the infecting agent so that it is no longer dangerous may be enough to turn it into a vaccine. In fact, this often makes a better vaccine; if the damaged organism continues to reproduce in the body, it provides a continuous stimulus to the immune system rather than a short-lived single one.

Now we should examine why vaccines might fail. First, you might fail to respond. This may be due to an immunological defect – some vaccines fail to work in HIV patients, for example, while other live vaccines may be dangerous in such a context. For some unknown reason some healthy people may be non-responders; this is sometimes encountered in vaccination for hepatitis B. There may be human error introduced into the process: wrong doses given; vaccine improperly stored; people failing to attend for boosters. Finally, the disease itself may be simply unsuitable for vaccine development.

TB falls into just such a category. The bacterium belongs to a group of organisms called mycobacteria. They are also known as acid- and alcohol-fast, because of their staining characteristics. They carry a tough, waxy outer coat. Indeed, it was the presence of this coat which made identification of the bacterium so difficult – the early stains simply failed to stick to the germ. The presence of this coat makes the bacterium oddly inert. It simply fails to generate a powerful immune response. This is one of the reasons it can lie dormant for so long; our immune systems practically ignore it. There is a further problem with TB: to control it effectively you need two vaccines, one to stop children acquiring the condition in the first place and the second to prevent reactivation of disease in people with latent infection. It isn't hard to see why the immune response you are seeking to invoke is different in each situation.

There are TB vaccines in development. One, called rBCG30, seeks to exploit the existing BCG vaccine. It works by using a harmless mutant strain which is engineered to produce one of the rather weak surface marker stimulants in larger concentrations. It is undergoing early trials as I write. There is a further technical difficulty with TB research, in that animal models are often unreliable as the human immune response is quite different to theirs. The best model is the guinea pig. While this does generate difficulties, they are as nothing when compared to the problems of developing an animal model for HIV infection, which I will outline below.

Scientific breakthroughs often occur when clever people make connections between apparently unrelated phenomena. Sometimes, though, the products of brilliant and mercurial minds prove just too challenging for the scientific community to accept. I performed my research in a laboratory at University College London full of such clever people. Professors John Stanford and Graham Rook were working on another TB vaccine. They found one, with novel and exciting methods of acting and wildly wider applications than would seem possible. Their work challenged much scientific orthodoxy.

Stanford and Rook drew a connection between a number of apparently disparate facts. It has long been known that patients with leprosy rarely develop TB. Leprosy is caused by a bacterium very like TB, also belonging to the mycobacteria group. TB also has a patchy distribution, not entirely explained by genetic susceptibility or regional social factors. Stanford and Rook knew also about the hypothesis which said that the variable response to BCG may be due to exposure to local harmless environmental mycobacteria (discussed more fully in Chapter Six). The conclusion they drew was that perhaps people who were exposed to certain mycobacteria derived immunity to TB, rather like the cross-immunity to leprosy only without the unpleasant consequences of suffering that disease.

They searched among likely candidates for such a harmless environmental organism, and found a likely candidate in a bug called *Mycobacterium vaccae*. They began to investigate a killed preparation of this germ as a TB vaccine, and in doing so they found something quite remarkable and unexpected. The effect on the immune system of even single doses was profound and persistent; it seemed to shift its whole axis. The nature of the switch is complex, but in essence the principle is this. White blood cells may be sub-classified according to the chemicals they produce. Some diseases – asthma, allergies, some cancers and TB – are characterised by a relative excess of white blood cells called lymphocytes producing chemicals that exacerbate these conditions. I will call this the Th2 state without further explanation. *M. vaccae* potently shifts the immune response to the opposite Th1 state. There are diseases characterised by an excess of Th1 chemicals, but the Th2 type are increasingly common. Stanford and Rook have therefore presented their product, SRL172 and its derivative SRP199, as treatment for a very wide variety of conditions, including asthma and cancers.

I was working with John and Graham when the results of a safety study into the effects of *M. vaccae* in TB patients were published.

They had previously formed a biotech company and floated it on the Stock Exchange. By the evening before those results were published, their share value had risen from the initial £1 to £12. Then something most peculiar happened. The study was, as I have said, an investigation into safety. It was compared with standard TB treatment which, when properly administered, is 90 per cent effective. Not surprisingly, *M. vaccae* did not improve on this. Suddenly, this study was presented as showing that *M. vaccae* did not work. The share price fell to 50p instantly.

This study effectively sank *M. vaccae* as a TB treatment. It is still occasionally used as an adjunct for disease in which all else is failing, where the bacterium is resistant to multiple drugs. But no venture capitalist is likely to finance research into a treatment whose efficacy has been questioned, particularly when the disease principally affects poorer countries. Nobody knows for certain whether *M. vaccae* works in TB. However, the science behind it is valid. The huge advantage of *M. vaccae* would have been its astonishingly low cost. It can almost be made in a kitchen, and costs mere pennies per dose.

The same problems of designing a vaccine for *Mycobacterium tuberculosis* and for diarrhoeal illnesses apply to another extremely unpleasant Quiet Killer. Meningitis is a disease with a vast number of causes. The clinical signs of meningitis were described in the Middle Ages. Francisco de Goya, the painter, may have been left deaf after suffering a bout in 1792. The disease was originally called 'spotted fever', because of the typical rash of some variants. The organism that has attracted the most attention in the developed world is probably that caused by the bacterium *Meningococcus*, or *Neisseria meningitidis*, which was not clearly described until 1884. This has a predilection for children and young adults. Untreated, it has 100 per cent mortality (which of course brings Goya's diagnosis into question). Such enormous strides have been made in vaccination for bacterial meningitis that I recently saw the question, 'Meningitis – a Vaccine Preventable Disease: Discuss' set in a postgraduate exam for microbiologists. Of course, this is a deliberately provocative question, but there are indeed effective vaccines for *Haemophilus influenzae* and *Streptococcus pneumoniae*, two of the commonest causes of vicious and sometimes fatal bacterial meningitis.

The situation with the *Meningococcus* bacterium is more complex, as it has more than one strain. These are defined by the presence of complex sugars on the outer coating of the bacterial cell. There are basically four strains, denoted by A, B, C and W137. The last of these is also known as the Haj strain, as it has caused outbreaks during religious pilgrimages to Mecca. There are effective vaccines for three of the four – A, C and Haj. However, the B strain has proven strangely unprepared to yield to vaccination. Its polysaccharides are rather like the waxy mycolic acids that make up the coat of *Mycobacterium tuberculosis* – oddly inert. At the same time, they are a moving target. Vaccines have been developed which seem to work in some countries but not others; there is a promising vaccine in development in New Zealand. There is a further theoretical hazard related to vaccination. The *Meningococcus* is capable of changing its polysaccharides; the concern was that vaccinating against A and C would allow B to replace them by creeping into a vacant ecological niche. Group B is already responsible for 65 per cent of meningococcal meningitis in some countries. Fortunately, this does not seem to be happening and the incidence of vaccine-preventable strains has fallen significantly in countries which have adopted it.

Physicians who have witnessed the astonishing rapidity of progression of meningococcal disease in young people observe the anti-vaccination lobby with rueful despair. I recall a medical student who told his friends he was returning to his hall of residence as he felt slightly unwell. Luckily, one of his mates went to check on him, and found him very ill indeed. In the period between being found and being carried to the casualty department – a distance of about 500 metres – the foul, florid purple rash of meningococcal septicaemia appeared on his skin, visibly sprouting new blotches as his friends desperately rushed him to assistance. He survived, but was left profoundly deaf.

The others in our list of problematic 'diseases that never went away' do not respond to vaccination for almost precisely the opposite reason. A feature of vaccination which should have become apparent is that it does not actually prevent infection. It alerts the immune system to the kind of markers – more correctly called antigens – that the invader might carry. When a real infection is met, the vaccinated immune response is swift enough to eradicate the invasion before it can cause severe disease. We have mentioned the extraordinary ability of some Quiet Killers to evade the immune system. The example I used was *Trypanosoma Brucei*, the agent of sleeping sickness, because it is such a master of disguise. The agent of the most lethal strain of malaria, *Plasmodium falciparum*, is capable of just the same sorts of tricks. Further, the markers on the surface of the parasite are present in huge and diverse numbers. They also vary during the complex life cycle of the infection, which has both sexual and asexual phases and takes place in different organs. The antigens present on the first invaders – the sporozoites – are different from those during the next phase – the merozoites – which emerge from the liver and burrow into the red blood cells. It is entirely possible to have mixed infections of more than one species and more than one strain. This Quiet Killer fights dirty.

There are four species of human malaria. Other species infect animals. Two of the human forms, *falciparum* and *vivax*, cause the vast majority of deaths, with *falciparum* by far the more dangerous. The disease is widespread in sub-Saharan Africa, and is common throughout tropical regions of China, India, South-East Asia, and South and Central America. Rather like *Meningococcus*, the disease causes most deaths and illness in the young. The majority of deaths from *falciparum* malaria occur in children under the age of 10, and the impact is especially severe in those under the age of 5. Untreated, up to 20 per cent of people infected with *falciparum* malaria will die. Accurate estimates of how many contract malaria and how many die are hard to verify, but the best figures suggest one million deaths in Africa alone each year, with 200 million episodes of illness. The problem with collecting the information is that many feverish patients are presumptively treated for malaria in poor areas with few diagnostic facilities; the diagnosis may or may not be correct. Even sick children who have parasites detected in their blood may have chronic disease and actually be ill from some other cause. Many deaths occur at home with no medical consultation.

There is little doubt that malaria is a very important disease which creates a huge burden for impoverished tropical countries. The situation is complicated further by the consummate ability of the parasite to become resistant to drugs. Simple measures may control the risk: nets impregnated with insecticide have been proven to reduce transmission, while avoiding mosquito bites is easily the most effective measure. Spreading oil on stagnant water to disrupt the breeding of mosquitoes also works, as does DDT.

There are hopeful signs for vaccine discovery. Inhabitants of malarial areas do develop immunity, even if this is transient. Malaria parasites have been deliberately injected into people with subsequent immunity developing. This seemingly foolhardy experiment was rendered safe by irradiating the parasites in advance so they could not reproduce. The huge panel of possible antigens – markers – that might invoke immunity has been analysed. About forty of these look very promising. Some vaccines have undergone field trials and have shown some benefit. A flamboyant Colombian doctor called Manuel Pattaroyo presented the world's first vaccine to the world in the 1990s among much fanfare; it is called SPf66 and is based on a cocktail of synthetic proteins, or antigens. It caused much controversy at the time, to the extent that his research was denounced in *The Lancet*.

A better vaccine should be financially feasible. There was a flurry of interest in prevention when about 100,000 American soldiers developed malaria during the Vietnam War, but the interest waned as they came home. Now the hunt is on again. The Bill & Melinda Gates Foundation announced a philanthropic $1 billion scheme in 1999 to develop vaccines for diseases in the Third World, malaria included. There has been further funding from the US National Institutes of Health, the World Health Organization and Britain's Wellcome Trust. Total pledged funds from all sources amount to more than $100 million. The World Bank has promised up to $500 million in interest-free loans to African countries for malaria prevention and control. The four-nation Roll Back Malaria Campaign has been attacking the disease on a variety of fronts since 1998, including vaccines, nets, sterilised mosquitoes and better disease mapping. It would be heart-warming to believe that all of this effort is purely altruistic. One cannot help thinking that the West Nile Virus experience must have concentrated the minds of many politicians. A novel Quiet Killer spreading uncontrollably across the United States, plus the threat of new diseases spreading due to global warming, whether correct or not, must have given some pause for thought. In an ironic twist, as if to emphasise the threat to the West, the director of the Bill & Melinda Gates Foundation malaria research programme, Regina Rabinovich, returned from a fact-finding mission to the Gambia and promptly fell ill with malaria.

HIV is discussed in Chapter Ten; it is worth mentioning again here while we are discussing vaccine development. This virus suffers from a further difficulty. We mentioned that the guinea pig provides the most reliable animal model for TB. Other diseases are even more particular – in leprosy, only the nine-banded armadillo provides a suitable comparator for human disease. Irrespective of your personal views on animal experimentation, it is very difficult indeed to develop a vaccine without an animal model. As yet, there has been no reliable animal model for HIV disease. Although other animals like cats and seals suffer from similar viral infections, and the best available theory suggests that HIV may be a mutated simian virus, the models available to us are just not close enough to depend upon. SIV – Simian Immunodeficiency Virus, which infects apes – is too different from HIV to compare properly. Chimpanzees can be infected with HIV, but the subsequent disease course in their case is not the same as in humans, which makes vaccine effects difficult to evaluate. Chimaeric viruses, hybrids of HIV and SIV, can be developed, but you can imagine the difficulties involved in interpreting the relevant results. There is some hope for a suitable animal model in the so-called transgenic (genetically modified) rat, but otherwise we are left with testing material derived from an incurable virus on human volunteers. Viral vaccines are not necessarily whole viruses, but how certain would you like me to be that there is no possibility of contamination with live virus in my preparation before I inject you? You might argue that we could conduct tests on people who already have HIV. Aside from the ethical issue here, how would you confirm your results? Supposing it went wrong, what are the effects of infection with two different viruses? Contamination with live virus has already occurred with rabies vaccination. Current advice is that live polio vaccine should not be given where there is a person with severely damaged immunity in the household, as wild-type polio transmission may result. How much more careful do we need to be with the AIDS virus?

The quest for a vaccine for HIV is, nevertheless, advancing – at least as far as HIV-1 is concerned (see Chapter Ten for an explanation of HIV-1 and -2). In Chapter Eleven, I discuss the concept of being 'target-rich, product-poor'. Sadly, this has been the experience with HIV vaccines to date. Nonetheless, I find these elegant approaches to new vaccines fascinating, and so include a few here. They are all at various stages of trial, either in humans or animals.

The most straightforward vaccine is also probably the most dangerous – the live, attenuated (damaged) virus, which is under investigation on primates. As may be imagined, the risk for humans is not small. The killed virus has also been tested. With this option, in addition to the risk of contamination with live virus, it is also technically difficult to produce in large enough quantities. Smashed-up particles or genetically produced facsimiles of the virus's protein envelope are under assessment; in one refinement, these can be attached to a harmless canarypox virus vector or mass-produced by other viruses. It is possible to genetically modify other harmless viruses to incorporate HIV genes. This has proved a fairly weak stimulus to immunity, and is complex to prepare. Even more demanding are replicons and pseudovirions. These are incomplete HIV-like particles that are deficient in their ability to reproduce. They nonetheless present the relevant 'markers' or antigens to the immune system. An easier challenge is the bacterium that is genetically modified to produce HIV proteins. Naked HIV DNA that encodes one or more HIV genes may stimulate the correct response. The concern here is that these genes may themselves cause some damage to human cells. Finally, a group from St George's Hospital, London, is experimenting with vaginal vaccines. These are designed to prevent entry of the virus through the tissues of the vaginal wall, which is the chief route of infection in heterosexual transmission.

All of these highly sophisticated and almost beautiful concepts suffer from further difficulties. The object is clearly to reduce the transmission of HIV. Without a reliable animal model, what tests do you apply that confirm the efficacy of your vaccine? There are clearly ethical issues involved with injecting your hypothetically effective, but possibly risky, vaccine into susceptible populations and waiting to see if they develop HIV or not. The solution to this is that scientists tend to use so-called 'surrogate markers' of immunity. A surrogate marker is, broadly, something we can measure that accurately represents something we cannot measure. A good example is measuring blood cholesterol. We cannot properly measure 'risk' of having a heart attack. However, because there is a statistical association between elevated blood cholesterol and heart disease, an abnormal blood test is taken to represent an increased risk of having a heart attack. The association may be statistically valid even if there is no proven cause-and-effect between the two, although clearly the association is more reliable if such a relationship exists. It is presently believed that the behaviour of a subset of white blood cells called T-lymphocytes represents the best surrogate marker for immunity to HIV. A key part of vaccine research has been developing a test of T-lymphocyte function which all scientists can agree on, and which works in every laboratory in precisely the same way.

We will meet influenza again in Chapter Seven. Most people know that there is a vaccine available for influenza, and the elderly, diabetics, dialysis patients and other groups with damaged immunity are advised to have the vaccine annually. Why don't we just vaccinate everyone and have done with it? The answer lies in the peculiar ability of the influenza virus to offer a doubly moving target. Its genetic construction changes a little bit every year, and then every so often it undergoes a major revamp. We will discuss this in more detail later. Recently the whole strategy of annual vaccination has been called into question anyway. It may not be effective.

So, rather wearily, I come to one Quiet Killer which has not gone away but should have done. This disease illustrates the final reason why vaccines fail. In those parts of the world where it remains a killer, this preventable disease continues its slaughter of children because there is neither the money nor the will to confront it. Meanwhile in the West, where it kills rarely, complacent populations for whom the infection is just a word in a newspaper are rejecting a safe and effective vaccine through misinformation and perversity. This disease is measles. There is no scientific foundation, I believe, for deciding not to vaccinate and thus letting this potential killer become rife again. Science may not have all the answers, but it has the best ones at the moment. If anyone has anything better, then bring it on and let's test it.

FOUR

Killers in Extremis
Diseases of war, famine, and other special circumstances

Societies faced with overwhelming pestilence tend to collapse, albeit temporarily. The writings of Defoe, Boccaccio and Pepys allude to the social disorder that accompanied the Black Death. We know also that the reverse is true. When social order breaks down, through war or natural disaster, the Quiet Killers follow in its wake. The Four Horsemen of the Apocalypse are an ancient mythical image, and like many myths it has an origin in reality. Pestilence hitches a ride with those other horsemen, famine and war. In Indonesia, the disease to be feared following the tsunami was tetanus. In Europe during and after the First World War it was typhus, then influenza. There are other, more obvious examples such as cholera. Still others are less to be expected. For example, there was an outbreak of Crimea–Congo haemorrhagic fever following the recent war in Afghanistan; the First Gulf War resulted in a spate of new diagnoses of a new variety of a condition called *Leishmania major* among American servicemen.

We saw in the introduction the disastrous consequences of the influx of a previously unknown illness – measles – into a previously unexposed community. Of course, the traffic of the Quiet Killers has not always been in one direction alone. When humans encroach on new environments, especially if they are not indigenous to the area, then new diseases may result. The story of the first of our diseases that belongs in the category of special circumstances is remarkable, filled with drama, duels and intrigue.

In the developed world, we think ourselves safe from many of the Quiet Killers because our lives are so protected. We have clean, safe, reliable water supplies. Many of the insects which transmit deadly illnesses either cannot survive in our climate or have been controlled. We have social order; effective public health protection; efficient vaccination programmes. The disease I intend to discuss arose in the West at a time when enlightenment about such matters was just burgeoning. It is ironic that it was our comparative health which made its victims susceptible; the particular circumstances of its coming are telling for our modern experience.

In Philadelphia in 1793, more than 10 per cent of the entire population died of a mysterious illness which caused jaundice, vomiting of black bile and uncontrollable bleeding. The disease had spread into North and South America and the Caribbean from the seventeenth century. Where these animals were present, the disease seemed also to be decimating the monkey population, while the city of Memphis, Tennessee almost had to be abandoned in the 1840s. Opinions were bitterly divided about the new pestilence: in 1740 in Jamaica, a furious row broke out between Drs Parker Bennett and John Williams over the cause of the disease. Bennett thought, incorrectly, that this was a variety of malaria called blackwater fever. In the ensuing duel, both died. Various treatments for the terrifying new illness were tried out of desperation – blistering, cupping, bleeding. Nothing seemed to work, a fact which remains true to this day as there is no proven effective treatment for this disease. It also spread to Europe. In 1800, Barcelona was struck by the infection and 1 in 6 people died. An outbreak in Haiti killed 23,000 French soldiers. The disease was variously known as 'Yellow Jack', 'Yellow Breeze' or 'Black Vomit'. Luckily, most of us will only ever encounter it through vaccine regulations for travel to endemic areas. Most people know it best as Yellow Fever.

This disease travelled from East to West, and the special circumstance that brought it was not war, or famine, but inhumanity – in the form of slavery. It is also the story of mankind's greed. Once again Cromwell, he who possibly died of malaria, plays a part through his bigotry and loathing of Catholicism. Finally, the resolution of the mystery surrounding the disease led to the triumphant completion of one of the world's greatest engineering feats.

Oliver Cromwell had sought to destabilise the Spanish (Catholic) influence on the Americas by seizing Caribbean islands. Aside from their strategic importance, these were fertile lands with dwindling native populations, decimated by diseases imported from the West, like measles. They were ripe for commercial exploitation by greedy European powers. In 1655, a British force of 7,000 men took Jamaica from the Spanish. Many of the other islands in the region were annexed, ceded by treaty or invaded during the following years.

The world had developed a sweet tooth by the seventeenth century. The principle sop for this craving was sugar cane; there were fortunes to be made from this luxury commodity. Most of the Caribbean islands and the lowlands of the adjacent South American mainland were rainforest; to grow the cane, this inconvenient vegetation had to be cleared. This meant a number of unpredictable and unstable events, from which our deadly scourge was to emerge. Massive deforestation made for a change in ecology for the local wildlife. The rainforest canopy was brought to ground level, and with it the insect population, including mosquitoes such as *Aedes aegyptii*, the Yellow Fever mosquito. Loss of predatory birdlife meant larger numbers of mosquitoes survived; loss of rainforest canopy brought the mosquitoes into contact with man; and loss of the usual monkey hosts meant that the mosquitoes were more likely to bite humans. Monkeys are the natural hosts of Yellow Fever. Unlike many other monkey viruses, this one readily transmits to humans.

The work of forest clearance and cane harvest was performed principally by slaves. Many of these were from West Africa, where Yellow Fever was also indigenous. Some of these slaves would have previously encountered the disease and were therefore immune. Paradoxically, then, it was the unexposed, healthy white settlers from sterile cold climates who were most at risk of the disease. Almost half of the original force sent by Cromwell to Jamaica died.

More importantly, the worldwide trade in slaves meant that ships containing a mixture of susceptible and immune individuals, with their attendant mosquitoes, were being shipped around the world in huge numbers. A ship entirely full of immune slaves would not have transmitted the virus, because it could not have survived in their bloodstream, but they provided blood meals to enhance the survival of *Aedes aegyptii*. All susceptible individuals aboard a ship might have died before reaching their destination, as sometimes happened. But as for a ship containing a mixture of both, it is hard to think of a more efficient means of spreading a disease to new regions. It was almost certainly one of these slave ships which took Yellow Fever to North America. The first epidemic of Yellow Fever in the Americas came in 1647, striking Barbados first and then Guadeloupe, St Kitts, Cuba, the Yucatán and the east coasts of Central America generally. It killed perhaps 20 to 30 per cent of the local populations, and another 250 years were to elapse before the illness had been properly controlled.

Yellow Fever is one of the most vicious of the Quiet Killers. It is a capricious viral disease with almost wantonly malign features. It belongs to the same family as Japanese Encephalitis and hepatitis C. Unlike in most infectious diseases, the first victims were often not the elderly and children, but men – who are disproportionately affected – in the prime of health. This results from a peculiarity of the *Aedes aegyptii* mosquito. In contrast to other mosquitoes, this insect is happy in an urban habitat with clean water cisterns and in bustling areas in cities where men go about their business.

Not all of the victims of Yellow Fever are affected similarly; some may only have a mild infection. The more severe illness begins with fever, nausea and general malaise, which may remit two to three days from the onset. At this moment, the victim may be, cruelly, convinced that they are getting better. Only then would the true horror of the symptoms emerge. Every orifice of the body may start to bleed, including the anus, eyes and sweat glands. Vomit may be black. There could be constant hiccupping, so that even relatively lucid moments provide no comfort. To the end, the victim may be convinced that he or she was recovering.

It was not until 1900 that the US military decided to tackle the problem. Gradually, small pieces of the jigsaw began to assemble. It had been known since 1802 that the disease was not transmissible through body fluids, when a physician called Firth swallowed the bloodstained vomit of a Yellow Fever victim and remained well. The military physician Walter Reed observed that, against prediction, soldiers in Cuba nursed in beds previously occupied by Yellow Fever victims did not all develop the disease. The notion that something else was spreading the disease led Drs Jesse Lazear and Aristide Agremont to experiment with mosquitoes. They deliberately permitted a colleague, Dr James Carroll, to be bitten by a mosquito. Agremont's account of the astounding and ground-breaking experiment survives, dated 31 August 1900. Carroll had started to show symptoms of Yellow Fever. The original narrative is reproduced here, because it is one of the most seminal in infectious diseases history, and also has a compelling immediacy. I would also ask you to reflect on the chances of this kind of experiment being repeated nowadays.

As the idea that Carroll's fever must have been caused by the mosquito that was applied to him four days before became fixed upon our minds, we decided to test it upon the first non-immune person who should offer himself to be bitten; this was of common occurrence and taken much as a joke among the soldiers about the military hospital. Barely fifteen minutes may have elapsed since we had come to this decision when, as Lazear stood at the door of the laboratory trying to 'coax' a mosquito to pass from one test-tube into another, a soldier came walking by towards the hospital buildings; he saluted, as it is customary in the army upon meeting an officer, but, as Lazear had both hands engaged, he answered with a rather pleasant 'Good morning.' The man stopped upon coming abreast, curious no doubt to see the performance with the tubes, and after gazing for a minute or two at the insects he said: 'You still fooling with mosquitoes, Doctor?' 'Yes,' returned Lazear, 'will you take a bite?' 'Sure, I ain't scared of 'em,' responded the man. When I heard this, I left the microscope and stepped to the door, where the short conversation had taken place; Lazear looked at me as though in consultation; I nodded assent, then turned to the soldier and asked him to come inside and bare his forearm. Upon a slip of paper I wrote his name while several mosquitoes took their fill; William E. Dean, American by birth, belonging to Troop B, Seventh Cavalry; he said that he had never been in the tropics before and had not left the military reservation for nearly two months. The conditions for a test case were quite ideal.

Dean developed Yellow Fever. By a quirk of fate, Carroll and Dean both survived, while Lazear himself died of the disease.

In the 1860s the huge Panama Canal project had ended in failure – not because of financial collapse or technical difficulty, but because so many labourers had been dying of Yellow Fever. In all, 52,816 died. US Army physician William Gorgas realised that the life-cycle of *Aedes aegyptii* could be disrupted in the pools of stagnant water where they bred. Their floating larvae need to breathe air through a siphon. Simply pouring on a layer of oil suffocated them. Thus the mosquitoes were destroyed and the Panama Canal was completed in 1913. A vaccine became available in 1935; cases of Yellow Fever are now extremely rare. Worldwide incidence is now officially recorded at between 1,000 to 3,000 per year, although this may be an underestimate.

Other Quiet Killers stalk war zones. As we saw in Chapter Three, diarrhoeal illnesses have wrought havoc on military campaigns. Although of the *Salmonella* family, typhoid is not usually a cause of diarrhoea except in its terminal stages, but causes death by septicaemia or perforation of the intestines. Like many other diseases, it is introduced to the body through food or water contaminated by faeces and thus is well adapted to ravage the unsanitary conditions of theatres of war. Soldiers introduced to an area where diseases are endemic will be even more prone than the local population, because they will have no immunological protection. Where they are endemic, malaria, Yellow Fever, sandfly fever and Ebola virus can decimate armies and refugee camps. Wound infections are of course common, and gangrene may result. Cholera is often mentioned during war and natural disasters like floods as a possible risk for epidemics. In fact, we are still within the seventh recorded cholera pandemic, which began in 1961 and is known as 'El Tor'; and this has had very little to do with war or disaster. The previous pandemics began in 1817 in India, spreading worldwide to include Europe and America, with New York being affected particularly badly. There have been five more pandemics since, and before El Tor. This is a variety of cholera that has changed its nature; paradoxically, it has been able to spread worldwide because it is actually less virulent than 'classical' cholera and therefore has more unwitting, apparently healthy carriers to transmit the infection. It is perfectly capable of killing, though. Cholera is an unpleasant disease characterised by profuse and watery diarrhoea; death is by dehydration and salt loss. El Tor also seems to be more robust and better able to survive in the environment than the variety it replaced. There was an outbreak among refugees on the India–Bangladesh border in 1971 during the War of Independence; however, this was within an area already affected by El Tor. Refugee movements may transmit cholera to previously uninfected areas, and hospital outbreaks in overcrowded areas beset by refugees have occurred. There is one misconception about cholera. It is often mentioned where floods have left corpses floating unrecoverably in rivers. Generally, this is not a source of the disease, unless the corpse was already a cholera victim or the river was already contaminated with cholera. The illness is caused by a specific bacterium. It cannot suddenly appear, even in a decaying body. The notion that a decomposing corpse might allow the disease to develop is dangerously akin to the long-discredited theory of spontaneous generation.

It was noted by military doctors during the Second World War that there was a massive disparity between the rates of infections in soldiers with gunshot wounds serving on different fronts. The victims shot in the warm North African campaign had a likelihood of infection different by a factor of three to the soldiers from the frozen zones of the Russian theatre. If you had thought that it was the warmer region, more conducive to bacterial growth, that had the higher rate of infection, then you should think again. It was among the gelid plains of the East that wound infections were so troublesome. The reason? Soldiers in North Africa often fought semi-naked because of the heat. A bullet would have dragged a thin layer of shirt at most behind it. In the frozen steppes, soldiers would wear multiple layers of clothing, often not changing or washing for weeks on end. Like it or not, in microbiological terms there is little to choose between the clothes that we wear and excrement.

The tendency of the Quiet Killers to thrive in conditions of war is partly explained by dislocated, malnourished migrating masses huddling to one another in unhygienic conditions – typhus is an excellent example, being spread by lice. There are other reasons, though, why war might ease the transmission of infectious diseases. I cite here two experiments from scientific literature which illustrate this point. Stressed mice are more likely to contract TB. Stressed deer are more likely to develop listeria. The method of stressing the animals was different in each experiment, although equally bizarre. The mice were subjected to 'restraint' stress – basically, they were allowed to see and smell their food for some of the day, but not eat it. The deer were made to travel contrary to their preferred direction of movement. Deer show a peculiarity in that in herds they like to move in a clockwise direction; make them move anti-clockwise and they become very stressed indeed. Stress is an excellent way of suppressing immunity; could there be a more stressful environment than a theatre of war? The hormone cortisol appears to be responsible; this is discussed in Chapter Three. Its effect is reflected in varying mortality rates for illnesses like typhus. Untreated, epidemic typhus has a mortality of 20 per cent. However, this may rise to 50 per cent under conditions of war and social dislocation. At the Siege of Granada in 1489, 17,000 died of typhus compared to 3,000 battle victims. On the Eastern Front in the First World War, delousing stations were set up to control the vector; nonetheless, 150,000 died in Serbia alone. The physician Girolamo Fracastoro offered one of the first and most accurate accounts of typhus in his 1546 book, *De Contagione et Contagiosis Morbis*: fever and fatigue followed by general prostration and delirium; then a general rash that looked like flea-bites or, in some cases, larger spots about the size of lentils, the most characteristic associated symptom. The disease itself is from the Greek 'typhos', meaning a fog, which derives from the clouded consciousness or delirium. Ricketts, the scientist after whom the *Rickettsiae* which cause typhus is named, died of it himself.

The attendant malnutrition of famine and crop failure are as suppressive to the immune system as cortisol. Starvation in fact induces a stress-like response where cortisol is produced to excess. Protein malnutrition, also known by the name kwashiorkor, incapacitates the white blood cells as effectively as chronic alcohol excess. The body needs, under conditions of fuel-starvation, to make emergency choices. There is a hierarchy of body systems which are protected above all others, particularly the brain, heart and lungs. Fat and muscle are combusted first, and immune cells fall about halfway up the pecking order. Thus, infections like measles and viral gastroenteritis exact a far higher toll under these circumstances. Drinking water may be scarce and contaminated with faecal bacteria. Dehydration reduces the capacity of the body to transport nutrients, and compounds the potentially fatal fall in blood pressure associated with many infections; failure of the kidneys allows accumulation of waste products that are toxic to white blood cells. Malnutrition may be compounded by worm infections in such unsanitary conditions. Common worm parasites then consume what little sustenance is available. The burden of an infectious disease adds further demands on a failing system. Chemicals – cytokines – produced in some infections speed the metabolic rate; some cause loss of appetite. Fever, to be sustained, requires energy. Deficiencies of vitamins lead to specific diseases such as scurvy, beriberi and pellagra, which permit other infectious agents to enter. A spiralling cycle of decline is commenced, each component exacerbating the others.

During the Great Irish Potato Famine of 1846–52 – itself caused by an infectious agent, the fungus *Phytophthora infestans* – the principal causes of death were infectious diseases such as typhoid, relapsing fever, dysentery and typhus. The last of these was so closely associated with deaths during this grim period of European history that it came to be known as Irish Famine Fever. It caused huge mortality among deliberately starved concentration camp inmates in the Second World War. Relapsing fever is a further louse-borne disease caused by bacteria similar to syphilis called *Borrelia recurrentis*; death is usually by shock. In excess of one million are believed to have died during the Irish Famine years, many in overcrowded disease-ridden ships. The political consequences of the famine are still with us, in the form of militant Irish nationalism and mass migration to the United States and other nations. Similar illnesses combined with malaria and tropical disease caused enormous mortality among Allied Prisoners of War and forced labourers in the Far East during the Second World War. Famine continues to menace certain parts of the globe, and the Quiet Killers still exact their toll where such disasters occur.

Paradoxically, the affluence and plenty of the developed world has led to an increase in infectious disease among the overfed. Obesity and its frequent consequence of diabetes both predispose to infections, often but not solely of the skin. There is also a worldwide epidemic of a condition called hepatic steatosis, where the liver becomes infiltrated with fat. The liver is intimately involved with immunity; inevitably, susceptibility to infectious agents will follow.

This is the grotesque irony at the heart of this book. While millions of the deprived and malnourished die of our old enemies such as measles, in the West we are making ourselves dangerously susceptible to the effects of otherwise trivial infections by our overindulgence, greed and lethargy. Before I move on to the diseases that our cultural enemies might wish to wreak on us in the form of bioterrorism, I will end with a final thought about the principal illnesses which kill in the privileged and overnourished. They are cancer, heart disease, stroke, chronic lung disease and diabetes. Every single one of these – including obesity – probably has at least one infectious component. In fact, of the ten leading causes of death in the United States, only one – accidents and violent death – has no known or postulated infectious element. The Quiet Killers are still having the last laugh.

FIVE

Agents of Infection
Diseases that someone might want to bring back

There is an ancient Chinese curse which says, 'May you live in interesting times'. Today, we live in just such times. Since 9/11 there has been something of a resurgence of anxiety in the concept of infectious illness as a tool of warfare. If aeroplanes, why not petri dishes? The Quiet Killers have enough opportunity to trouble us, you might think, without our making it easy for them. There are, though, some who would invoke their power for their own ends. The world has begun, with reason, to fear deliberate release of infectious agents as never before. The reality of using germs for warfare is nothing new. Sadly, ever since humankind discovered the use of tools, then just about anything that might fall within reach has served as a weapon. Infectious diseases have been no exception. There is no monopoly of the moral low ground as far as bioterrorism is concerned, either. The ancient Greeks were just as guilty as the most inhumane modern terrorist cell; bioterrorism has been repeatedly recorded on the North American continent, and in the modern era.

There is something peculiarly chilling about the ability to harness the Quiet Killers to evil purpose. Partly this must be due to their invisibility, and the stealth with which they attack. Partly also it must be due to their lack of discrimination: the babe-in-arms and the grandparent are as much a target as the soldier. But as much as anything, we must fear bioterrorism for ancient, atavistic reasons. As the reader will be aware from earlier chapters, the Quiet Killers have stalked humans since the earliest times. Indeed, humankind may owe much of its evolution to the challenges posed by infection – the so-called Red Queen hypothesis is discussed in Chapter Six.

However, the appearance of an outbreak of a particular constellation of symptoms – say, rash, fever, headache, perhaps followed by death – must have seemed more terrifying than ravening wolves to early humans, more so for being less explicable. No wonder, then, that spirits were invoked to explain such illnesses; until well into the nineteenth century some infectious diseases were perceived as divine punishment.

For a while, as we know, we seemed to have infectious diseases vanquished. Our metaphorical campfire glowed brightly enough to scare away the circling djinns. Those fires may now be dying down a little. The growing realisation that the tide seems to be turning in favour of infectious diseases feeds our anxieties; how much more bitter that our enemies should taunt us with weapons from another battle that we are already losing?

If you had to design an imaginary weapon of terrorism, you might make your choice from the following list of the qualities you needed from it. It should be cheap and not technologically too demanding to produce. It should be easily transportable across international borders without detection. Its effects should make obvious the terrorist nature of the assault, for which you can claim responsibility. It should be controllable: the first attack should kill enough people to cause dismay, but not so many that there is no one left to terrorise. The implication of the attack should be that it could be repeated on a much larger scale, with far more casualties. Ideally, the fear of the weapon should be enough to help you to make your demands without ever having to prove that it actually works. The Quiet Killers fulfil all these criteria, especially the last.

In a sense, there is no difference between death by bullet and death by germ. Indeed, until relatively recently a soldier was more likely to die of the effects of an infected wound, or of infection acquired off the battlefield, than of damage from the bullet itself. But, for reasons outlined above, terror does not work exclusively by mass slaughter. It works by fear. Understanding the nature of the germs of terror can reduce that fear. This chapter will examine some of the history of bioterrorism, and look at the individual agents. Are our fears justified?

The first documented evidence of a bioterrorist attack is of one that occurred in the sixth century BC, when the Assyrians poisoned the wells of their enemies the Persians with ergot. This is an alkaloid poison which is derived from rye grain contaminated with the fungus *Claviceps*. Ergot poisoning is particularly unpleasant, leading to gangrene of the fingers, toes and limbs. Mass ergot poisoning has undoubtedly occurred throughout history, being so common at one time that it was given its own folk name – St Anthony's fire. Pilgrimages to the shrine of St Anthony, in the *Claviceps*-free Swiss Alps, led to the disease being cured. Some believe hallucinogenic ergot may have caused the strange behaviour of women in Salem, Massachusetts that led to the Salem witch trials of 1692. Ergotism is an unlikely means of modern terror plots as rye is no longer used as a major food source in western societies; producing enough contaminated rye to present a serious threat to human health, except on a very small scale, would require agricultural quantities of cereal production.

Industrially produced synthetic ergot alkaloids are, however, available and used pharmaceutically. Poisoning depends on dosage; it is not a reliable toxin. It will not be considered again in this chapter, except to mention controversy from a related poison derived from fungi called T2, a trichothecene mycotoxin. During the late 1970s, there were reports from Laos and Cambodia of helicopter and plane attacks, spraying aerosols of several colours. Exposed people and animals became disorientated and ill. Some died. These attacks were known as 'Yellow Rain'. These may or may not have been biological warfare agents: some have argued – not very convincingly – that they were really the faeces of passing swarms of bees. Similar attacks may have occurred in Afghanistan in the 1970s and 1980s.

*   *   *

The Black Death itself may have been a consequence of biological warfare. In 1346, the Tatar Army was laying siege to the city of Kaffa, on the Crimea, now known as Theodosia. The Tatars are believed to have catapulted their diseased dead over the walls of the city; plague followed inevitably. The surrender was thus forced, although casualties were so appalling on the Tatar side that the siege was lifted anyway. Those infected who then fled from Kaffa – in particular, a company of Italian merchants who were trapped in the siege – may well have been the source of the ensuing plague pandemic which killed 24 million people. Between a half and a third of the population of Europe died; the infection alternated between being endemic and epidemic throughout Europe for the next 300 years. Thousands of cases still occur in Africa each year. The Italian merchants sailed to Genoa; plague is said to have broken out there the day after their ship docked. The theory does beg several questions. How did the plague infect the Tatars in the first place? How was this different from the reports of what was almost certainly plague in Europe in Roman times, for example the Plague of Justinian in AD 540–90? Why did the disease only break out the day after the Genoese merchants landed, when the incubation period is 2–5 days (maximum, 15). Nonetheless, the theory makes biological and temporal sense. The association between warfare and infectious disease has been a cursed duet throughout history, even without the deliberate intervention of humans.

The practice of hurling plague-infected soldiers over the walls of besieged cities has been repeated on several occasions through history. During the Battle of Carolstein in 1422, Lithuanian soldiers added insult to injury by catapulting 2,000 cartloads of excrement over the castle walls as well as the bodies of their plague-ridden soldiers. The Russians troops practised similar methods in 1710 and 1718, by hurling plagued corpses over the city walls of Reval during wars with Sweden.

Between 4 June 1796 and 2 February 1797, Napoleon Bonaparte laid siege to the city of Mantua, the crucial episode in his first Italian campaign; his aim was to exclude Austrians from northern Italy. The city was easy to besiege: the only access to it was via five causeways over the Mincio river. However, he was repeatedly attacked by relieving Austrian soldiers. In an effort to force the surrender, he supposedly attempted to infect the city with 'swamp fever'. The details beyond this are a little unclear. Swamp fever may be either leptospirosis – Weil's disease, an infection carried by rats – or malaria. Neither would be a very effective bioterrorism agent – although malaria may have been used in more modern times, as we shall see. Although both leptospirosis and malaria are potentially lethal, and they may have caused terror among the besieged, they fail some of our criteria of useful biological weapons. Indeed, Napoleon's ultimate victory over the Austrians was purely military.

A more suitable bacterium for use as a weapon is *Burkholderia pseudomallei*. This is responsible for the condition known as glanders in horses. In humans, it causes an extremely unpleasant, even fatal disease called melioidosis. It was first described among drug addicts in Yangon, Burma in 1912, and it continues to kill injecting drug users in South-East Asia to this day. Over 400 American and French soldiers contracted melioidosis during the Vietnam War. It was strongly suspected that German agents working in the United States deliberately infected cavalry horses and cattle that were to be shipped to the Western Front during the First World War.

The Japanese paid considerable attention to biological warfare, especially during the Sino-Japanese War of 1937–45. They constructed a research facility called Unit 731 in Pingfang, near the city of Harbin in occupied Manchuria, part of the puppet state of Manchukuo. It was under the leadership of General Ishii. Unit 731 was disguised as a water purification unit. Over 3,000 Chinese, Korean and Allied POWs were killed in there, as well as many more in field experiments. There are no absolutely accurate figures, but it is known that almost 1,000 post-mortems were carried out on the victims of biological warfare testing, mostly on people exposed to anthrax. By the end of the war, the Japanese had stockpiled 400kg of anthrax and had designed a bomb to disperse it. Unit 731 was not the only one of its type. The name serves as a generic term for other Japanese units, including Unit 543 (Hailar), Unit 773 (Songo unit), Unit 100 (Changchun), Unit 1644 (Nanjing), Unit 1855 (Beijing), Unit 8604 (Guangzhou) and Unit 9420 (Singapore). The units were not simply for research, either. Infected fleas were dropped over Manchuria in 1940 and an epidemic of plague followed. These units were destroyed after the war, and the 'scientists' who ran them were granted amnesty by the Americans.

The American biological warfare unit was established at Camp Detrick in Maryland in 1943. The Allies in London were then being regularly struck by rockets launched from German-occupied Europe. It was thought that these high-explosive rockets might easily be converted into efficient weapons for massive biological warfare attacks. Production of such agents eventually included *Bacillus anthracis*, botulinum toxin, *Francisella tularensis*, *Coxiella burnetii*, Venezuelan equine encephalitis virus, *Brucellus suis* and staphylococcal enterotoxin B. The programme was discontinued by executive order of President Richard M. Nixon in 1969, and the stocks were destroyed in the presence of suitably qualified independent witnesses. A defence programme designed to protect from biological warfare continues to exist.

Did the Nazis use malaria as a vehicle of biological terror? One historian claims so: in his book *The Conquest of Malaria: Italy, 1900–1962*, Professor Frank Snowden of Yale claims that during the autumn of 1943 German entomologists deliberately arranged the release of malaria-infected mosquitoes into the marshes between the Allied landing sites at Anzio and Rome. They prepared the site by reversing the pumps which drained the marshes. The scheme was masterminded by Erich Martini, a friend of Himmler. It would have been known that malaria is no respecter of the Geneva Convention; civilians would have been affected just as severely as soldiers. The Germans cared little about this, and were happy to punish the Italians who had changed sides by this moment. In the event, precisely this may have happened. The British and American troops were issued with anti-malarial medication and were protected. There were huge casualties on both sides following fierce fighting at Anzio, but not from malaria. Among the civilian population, matters were quite different. In 1943, 1,217 malaria cases were recorded in the area. In 1944, there were 54,929 cases. Malaria was not eradicated in the area until the 1950s, when the marshes were drained once again.

The world has made some attempt to face up to the horrors it has created in these grotesque weapons. The Biological Weapons Convention – more correctly known as the Convention on the Prohibition of the Development, Production and Stockpiling of Bacteriological (Biological) and Toxin Weapons and on their Destruction – was signed in 1972 by Britain, the United States, and many other countries. The convention explicitly outlaws the stockpiling of bioweapons and research into their development. Whether or not the signatories, which included Iraq, have abided by the convention is debatable.

There is no doubt that the Iraqis had an advanced bioweapons programme at least until 1995. They researched and developed weapons in the form of anthrax, botulinum toxins, *Clostridium perfringens*, aflatoxins and ricin. Field trials were conducted and a number of systems for delivering the poisons were explored, including rockets, aerial bombs and spray tanks. United Nations weapons inspectors noted in December 1990 that they had filled 100 R400 bombs with botulinum toxin, 50 with anthrax, and 16 with aflatoxin. There were also 13 Al Hussein (Scud) warheads filled with botulinum toxin, 10 with anthrax, and 2 with aflatoxin. In total, Iraq produced 19,000 litres of concentrated botulinum toxin (10,000 litres prepared in warheads); 8,500 litres of concentrated anthrax (6,500 in warheads); and 2,200 litres of aflatoxin (1,580 litres in warheads). On 2 August 1991, members of the Iraqi government confessed to leaders of United Nations Special Commission Team 7 that they had conducted research into the offensive use of *Bacillus anthracis*, botulinum toxins and *Clostridium perfringens* (gangrene) toxin. No previous government had confessed openly to research and development of biological weapons. The research facilities were based at Salman Pak and other sites, many of which were destroyed during the First Gulf War. Despite well-publicised suspicions, no evidence of research or development of biological weapons was unearthed after the Second Gulf War.

The former Soviet Union also signed the 1972 convention. In 1978, a Bulgarian agent called Georgi Markov was queuing for a bus. As he did so, he felt a sudden agonising pain in his calf. He turned to see a stranger carrying what seemed to be an umbrella. Markov died several days later. The 'umbrella' was in fact a pellet gun. The pellet, recovered post mortem, contained the deadly poison ricin. Although this toxin does not technically belong among the Quiet Killers, it is indubitably a bioweapon. It is extracted from by-products of castor oil production, from castor beans. It transpired that the assassination was carried out by the Bulgarian government. The ricin and umbrella were supplied by the Russians.

In April 1979, seven years after the Biological Weapons Convention, a city called Sverdlovsk, also known as Ykaterinberg, site of the massacre of the Romanovs, unexpectedly found itself in the grip of a horrible scourge. People in part of the city developed sudden difficulty in breathing, and many died shortly afterwards. Rumours at the time put the death toll at anywhere between 200 and 1,000. The terrified townspeople couldn't help noticing that all of the deaths had something in common. They all appeared to happen among people living south of the top secret Soviet Military Compound 19. The Ministry of Health blamed contaminated meat; nobody believed them. For years, rumour and counter-rumour surfaced and resurfaced. The nature of the outbreak and the fact that all the victims were downwind of the Military Compound, known to be a microbiology laboratory, fuelled suspicion that this was an accidental release into the air of something deadly that was being cooked up inside. These suspicions were confirmed in summer 1992. Boris Yeltsin, then President of Russia, confessed that the incident had indeed been a terrible accident involving release of a bioweapon. That weapon was anthrax.

Yeltsin said that he would terminate the former Soviet Union's Bioweapons Programme. Whether he did or not is debatable. Defectors from Russia, including a senior bioweapons programme manager called Ken Alibek, suggest that there was still a 'healthy' programme of research into biological warfare up to 1992, when he left. The programme included attempting to engineer bacteria and viruses into more lethal forms, by manipulating their genes or hybridising them with other bugs. Making them resistant to the usual antibiotics was also being attempted. Whether the Russian programme was reduced in scale, or terminated, depending on whom you believe, there was suddenly a glut of highly skilled but unemployed scientists available for hire. Some believe that these scientists may have taken some very grubby shillings indeed. The knowledge and training required to handle and manufacture bioweapons may spread and disseminate rather like the bacteria themselves. The Iraqis were said to have sent some bioweapons experts to Libya in 1998 to help with their fledgling bioweapons programme in Tripoli.

The problem with all biological agents, if you are going to use them for anything other than mass panic, is one of delivery systems. They may work fairly well in sieges, such as the Siege of Kaffa, where populations are trapped. If you are like Saddam Hussein once was, and have total control of a region, then you can send crop-sprayers to shower sarin or anthrax over your immobile target population. Under those circumstances, it also works pretty well as a weapon of genocide. There was some suggestion that the 9/11 pilots showed an unhealthy interest in crop-sprayers; in the immediate aftermath of the jet attacks on the World Trade Center, all such aircraft were grounded. Mounting a logistics operation like that over a western city would, now, be virtually impossible.

We should put the threat from biological weapons into context. Attempts to unleash biological Armageddon on civilian populations so far have been remarkable for their ineffectiveness. In 1995, it was reported that on at least ten occasions the Japanese Aum Shinrikyo cult had attempted to disperse anthrax, botulinum toxin, Q fever and Ebola against the population of Tokyo. Nobody noticed. What about the Sverdlovsk incident? The spores of this weaponised anthrax had been allowed to escape through the chimney of the military compound. As they escaped they formed a deadly plume, carried by the wind over the unsuspecting citizens. The episode was eventually analysed by an American team, led by a scientist called Meselson, who published their findings in one of the world's most reputable journals – *Science*. They identified 77 affected patients, 66 of whom died. All of them lived in a narrow band south of the military laboratory. The prevailing winds were from the north. Compare this figure to the 200 to 1,000 rumoured to have died by the citizens of Sverdlovsk. The first conclusion you might draw is how effective an agent of terror anthrax was; the rumours were up to thirty times the truth. The second is that as an actual killer, anthrax is not really that effective. Hundreds of thousands of people lived south of Military Compound 19. Only 66 died, despite the release of somewhere between 30g and 60g of anthrax spores – literally billions of them; not even simple anthrax spores either, but deliberately 'weaponised'. This means the particles were finely milled to make them smaller and easier to inhale. The most notable feature of these agents is that, compared with crashing an airliner into a skyscraper, they just don't cut it.

As we know, that was not the last time anthrax was used deliberately as an agent of terror. In the autumn of 2001, there were four cases of confirmed anthrax in the United States, one of which was a seven-month-old child. The method of delivery was the US postal service.

This episode had a consequence for me as a clinician which bordered on the comic. In 2001, I was working in an infectious diseases department in London. Anxiety about anthrax was high. We had several 'white powder' incidents in the hospital itself; these referred to members of the public finding white powder of any description and reporting them to the authorities as possible anthrax. A local elderly lady was sent some fragrant talcum powder by her sister in Florida. She gingerly presented the envelope to us, requesting that we test the white powder inside for anthrax. Furthermore, every skin lump, boil, scratch or bump was referred to our department as a possible anthrax case.

Then, one day, we were asked to see one patient whose story was more disturbing. He worked in the media, for an American company. He was a personal friend of one of the intended victims in New York who really had been sent anthrax powder in the post. He said he felt a little unwell, a few days after receiving an anonymous package containing white powder and some hard-core pornography. We examined him very thoroughly and found nothing to worry us;

nevertheless, we knew that pulmonary anthrax may have an incubation period, and so kept him under observation. We also arranged for blood tests to be sent to the correct laboratory, at the Centre for Applied Microbiological Research in Porton Down.

What many people do not realise about blood tests is that it is far harder to make them accurate for a rare disease than it is for a common one. Most tests give a numerical value, which you then have to compare with values among people you know to be negative for the disease. This allows you to determine the cut-off between positive and negative. A disease like anthrax is so rare that it is not a simple task to determine where the cut-off should be. The tests performed for anthrax include antibodies against three toxins produced by the bacterium. These are called Protective Factor, Oedema Factor and Lethal Factor. Late one afternoon, the lab at Porton Down rang us to say that our patient tested initially positive for one of these three, but for the reasons above, and without the confirmation of the other two, they did not know how to interpret the result. If only it had been Protective Factor which had been positive; I can't tell you how uncomfortable you feel having to explain to your terrified patient, 'Your anthrax test is positive for Lethal Factor. But don't worry about it.' Fortunately, this patient never became unwell and all of his subsequent tests were negative.

America holds the record for the largest peacetime bioterrorist assault so far. In 1984, locals in the town of The Dalles, Oregon began to notice bouts of unexplained illness. There seemed to be an epidemic of diarrhoea and vomiting in their midst. In total, 751 people were eventually affected. Some blamed the newcomers among them, the mysterious and secretive new sect of 4,000 people who had moved in nearby. They were trying to expand their premises on their 64,000-acre plot of land in Wasco County, a few miles from The Dalles. The state health authorities refused to accept the rumours, blaming faulty food handling. How very wrong they were . . .

The Dalles is a town with a population of about 20,000 on Interstate 84, near the edge of the Columbia river. Because of its position near the Interstate Highway, the town has many restaurants

– in 1984, 35, to be exact. The cult who had set up there were followers of Bhagwan Shree Rajneesh. The Rajneeshees had been refused planning permission for an extension to their premises by the Bureau of Land Management. When the State elections for State Commissioners came around, the 4,000 cult followers calculated that if everyone else in their county was too ill to vote, then they could gerrymander the result and overturn the decision that had gone against them.

The geographical location of The Dalles, and its many restaurants, worked well to the Rajneeshees' advantage. The cult had its own medical laboratory. It was a fairly simple matter to acquire and propagate cultures of *Salmonella typhimurium*, a cause of potentially lethal food poisoning. The cult, in addition to its own jets, helicopters and police force, had registered itself as a Medical Foundation and was able to obtain the cultures without challenge. Its members then set about spreading the bacterium into the town's salad bars and coffee creamers.

After prevarication, delay and evasion by the nervous state health authorities, the plot was finally investigated by the Oregon Attorney General, Dave Frohnmayer. He and his team uncovered vials of *Salmonella typhimurium* in the cult's lab. The strain turned out to be indistinguishable from that found in the food poisoning victims. There was some evidence of a plot to kill eleven Oregonians, including a local newspaper reporter. The FBI are also said to have found experimental cultures of the AIDS virus.

The most astonishing feature of this story is the treatment meted out to its hero, local Congressman Jim Weaver. He refused to accept the State Health Authority's initial version of events, that this was defective food-handling. His subsequent investigation did not make him popular: he was accused of racism and spat on by students when he visited the University of Oregon, and he was vilified in the local press. At the time, the episode received almost no publicity outside Oregon State. However, the events of 9/11 has concentrated the minds of many, and caused them to reflect on the bizarre events of seventeen years before. It has now passed into medical and political history.

What punishment was meted out to the culprits? Rajneesh was captured trying to flee. He was fined $400,000. His two henchwomen, 'Ma' Sheela and 'Ma' Puja, who performed the necessary scientific work, were extradited from West Germany to California and each served four years of a 24-year prison term. Bhagwan Shree Rajneesh died in 2000, a free man.

Other unconventional terrorist attacks have been more successful. There was, of course, the infamous poison-gas attack on the Tokyo underground. Although not technically an episode involving the Quiet Killers, it shows some of the technical difficulties of getting such agents into places where they can do harm. It was performed by a group who were no strangers to biological warfare – the Aum Shinrikyo cult, who had so signally failed with anthrax, botulinum, and so on. Twelve people died in the gas attack and, at the time of writing, more remain ill. In a grotesquely elegant manoeuvre, the terrorists unleashed the poison by placing plastic bags containing sarin on the floor of the train carriages, then piercing the lids with sharpened umbrella tips as they stepped off.

Observant readers will have noticed a glaring omission from the bioterrorist's armamentarium. I have left this until last because it is in a league of its own. We have already encountered it under the heading, 'Diseases that have gone away'; if it were not for this ghastly possible usage, it would be at one with the Bloody Flux in being consigned to history. Unlike all the other agents, this one is spread from person to person, turning everyone infected into a weapon. It is virulently infectious with a high mortality among the unvaccinated, which means almost anyone born after about 1970. Vaccine protection wanes with age. The disease may go undiagnosed while infectious because the initial symptoms may be mild. One infected individual could, in theory, spread the disease through an airport and contaminate much of the world within a few days. Experts disagree on the likely mortality, but it could – if not properly controlled – run into millions. The agent is smallpox.

The great paradox of smallpox is that the very fact of its eradication makes it all the more effective as a tool of warfare. The last natural cases of smallpox occurred in the 1970s; bar a laboratory accident detailed elsewhere, there have been no endemic cases in the western world since long before – the last major European outbreak was in former Yugoslavia in 1972. Outbreaks in Britain in the 1960s were imported. Nor was smallpox uniform in its effects. There were in fact three forms: *Variola major*, the most severe variant (see Chapter Two). Then there was varioloid, or modified disease, either following inoculation with Jenner's vaccine or variolation. Finally there was *Variola minor*, which is often known by its Brazilian name, 'alastrim'. This is a much milder illness than classical *Variola major*. It is caused by a slightly mutated version of the *Variola major* virus. Its victims were often not very ill; indeed, the condition was often misdiagnosed as chickenpox or measles. It has a mortality of about 1 per cent, although this is a historical figure derived from populations in which smallpox and alastrim were endemic. Nonetheless, people with alastrim often went about their business without seeking medical advice, and the illness spread easily.

Immunity to smallpox can arise from exposure to any of these forms. That immunity is of uncertain duration, but is probably lifelong in most instances. Consider, then, three populations. Number one was the historical population of Europe, with endemic alastrim and occasional epidemic smallpox; small numbers may have been partly protected by the dangerous process of variolation whereby matter from alastrim victims was inoculated into the healthy. While epidemics may have had a high proportional mortality, a significant proportion of the population would have had natural immunity; pandemics were therefore rare. This was the European situation from about the tenth century, until the arrival of Jesty, Woodville and Jenner in the eighteenth. The next population is the fully vaccinated community. Smallpox vaccination was compulsory in Britain until 1946; however, even so universal, 100 per cent coverage was never attained. The disease was eradicated in any case, for reasons outlined in Chapter One. In this highly protected population, epidemics could not occur. Occasional small outbreaks might arise from imported cases coming into contact with the small number of people in whom vaccination was missed, or was rejected for medical or other reasons, or had failed. This was the situation until the 1970s, when smallpox vaccination was abandoned. The third group would be the totally unexposed and unvaccinated population. We only need look to history to observe the catastrophic consequences of smallpox in this group. Populations with no natural or artificial immunity to Quiet Killers are peculiarly susceptible to them. So it was with measles in the South Pacific, when first western man visited, and so it was with smallpox among the Amerindians. This would be the case with the West now, among almost all populations born after vaccination was abandoned. Such people have neither natural nor artificial immunity.

Smallpox is a tried and tested biological weapon. Francisco Pizarro, the first of the Spanish conquistadors, is said to have presented South American natives with variola-contaminated clothing in the fifteenth century. Indeed, much of the legendary invincibility of the conquistadors may refer to their relative resistance to smallpox, compared to the previously unexposed Incas; certainly, when Cortés entered the Aztec capital of Tenochtitlan (modern Mexico City), to which he had laid siege, he found whole households filled with the bodies of smallpox victims. During the French and Indian War of 1754–67 in Canada, Sir Jeffrey Amherst gave blankets laced with smallpox to Indians loyal to the French during the siege of Fort Carillon. The stroke was effective: the fort rapidly fell. But the disease halved the local Indian population during the following years.

Supposing terrorists were to release smallpox, how effective would it be? The magnitude of any outbreak, whether terrorist-induced smallpox or mumps among university students, depends on three things: the number of people directly infected by the index case, known as the first-generation cases; the speed at which measures are introduced to control the case; and the R0, the number of secondary cases arising from each infected individual. If the R0 figure is less than 1, epidemics will end. As has been discussed, all that was needed to eradicate natural smallpox was to ensure that R0 was significantly and persistently less than 1, rather than vaccinating every single person. Of course, where R0 is greater than 1 for a prolonged period, then outbreak control becomes far harder.

To estimate R0 in the event of a terrorist attack, statisticians have examined figures from history and made guesses about how much immunity persists in the community. This is a controversial issue. Some say the figure is only 1.5; others greater than 20. Let us accept the broad consensus of an R0 of 5 for the community at large. Hospitals, where cases would be concentrated and airborne infections transmit easily, would tend to amplify the infection; an R0 figure of 10 in hospitals is generally agreed. These figures would mean a relatively slow development of the initial phases of an epidemic. Bringing it under control would therefore rely on the second of our conditions for rate of infectious disease transmission – the speed at which control measures are instigated.

We know this from Britain's foot-and-mouth epidemic among cattle in 2001; many other lessons about controlling a deliberate smallpox epidemic may be learned from that sorry episode. There was delay in confirming the diagnosis in the initial outbreak. There was also confusion and bitter argument about the R0 number, and how to handle the epidemic – by ring cull or vaccination. Of course, there would be no such argument about vaccination for smallpox; one would hope that no modern government would consider a ring cull. The Jenner/Jesty/Woodville vaccine has been around for two hundred years. However, it has to be remembered that smallpox vaccination is not entirely safe; in some outbreaks, mortality from vaccination was almost as high as mortality from wild smallpox. In 1962, smallpox was imported into Britain from Karachi. More than six million people were vaccinated as a consequence. There were sixty-two cases and twenty-four deaths. Nearly as many died from vaccination. It is unlikely that any medicines licensing authority in the western world would countenance the licensing of such a dangerous vaccine today.

Besides, what *is* the smallpox vaccine? We have already seen that smallpox was probably not eradicated by Jenner's cowpox vaccine, but by a hybrid virus whose origins are speculative at best. There are two vaccines available worldwide, and there is debate about which is better – the British (Lister) or American (New York City Board of Health) vaccine. It may not matter; if the rumours that the Russians were able to modify the virus to be no longer susceptible to vaccination are correct, neither may work.

Is a smallpox attack likely? It is no coincidence that the Rajneeshees used *Salmonella typhimurium*, while the Aum Shinrikyo cult attempted to use anthrax, botulinum toxin, Q fever and Ebola. Getting hold of these agents is far easier because people are still catching them. The Rajneeshees bought their salmonella from a catalogue. Smallpox is, officially, kept at only two sites. The first is in Atlanta, Georgia and is the Center for Disease Control and Prevention. The other is in Koltsovo, in the Novosibirsk region of Russia, and is the State Research Center of Virology and Biotechnology. The latter is more commonly known by the James Bond-ish title 'Vector'. Nobody is really certain how secure stocks have been at that site. The defector Ken Alibek tells us that the Russians cannot account for their smallpox stocks as to whether or not they have modified them to overcome vaccine immunity. Did the Iraqis have any? We will probably never know. But the West is taking the threat seriously. A smallpox rapid-reaction team has being created in Britain, and a vaccine – possibly the wrong one – is being stockpiled.

A smallpox attack would cause panic. Mass vaccination would be demanded, and politicians would find such calls very difficult to resist. So vaccination must be targeted. Just as important is the availability of rapid diagnostic facilities. Electron microscopy played a vital role in the laboratory escape outbreaks of the 1970s. For speed of response once suspicion is raised, it is just as important today. But the UK's machines are decaying fast; most are at least twenty years old. Microscopists used to keep their hand in by examining quality control samples sent from London, but this service stopped years ago. We also have to remember that all the smallpox hospitals closed long ago, and that the immunity of the well-vaccinated staff who worked there – if any are still alive – will have waned to virtually nothing. Let us hope that the lessons both of BSE, in which for nearly a decade policy was driven by the assumption that the probability of people being infected was 'remote', and of foot-and-mouth disease are being heeded. In the latter the contingency plan was designed for an outbreak of ten cases among susceptible animals yet before the first diagnosis was made there had been at least 57, and by the end 2,023.

The major current terrorist threat is said to be al-Qa'eda. So why wouldn't they use smallpox? Who knows? Maybe they don't have any. My guess is that they baulk at the Pyrrhic nature of such a stroke – Jeddah and Islamabad would be affected just as much as New York and London. Perhaps even bin Laden has qualms about the indiscriminate slaughter of his own. Let's hope so.

SIX

Beneficial Bugs?
Diseases that are good for us

The title concept may seem counter-intuitive, but there are, in fact, infections that can be beneficial to us. Infections acquired through vaccination are excluded from this category. Many vaccines are, of course, infectious agents that either have been modified to make them less dangerous, or are harmless close relatives of real killers like smallpox. These are discussed elsewhere in the book. Also excluded, for two reasons, are infections which we survive and to which we subsequently become immune, like measles. The first reason is that although such infections provide the benefit of long-term resistance to the disease, they do so at a risk. Measles is a disease with considerable mortality and a particularly vicious mode of death. Second, the development of long-term immunity to such infections is a predictable consequence which is common to many similar diseases. There are, though, other infections which appear to be highly beneficial to man, and indeed to many higher animals; and these are highly engrossing.

The people of Latvia, Lithuania and Estonia on the Baltic Sea and the people of Sweden have a great deal in common. Apart from years of shared history – Sweden even briefly ruled parts of the other Baltic States during that country's brief empire – the citizens of these nations have similar ethnic ancestry. Until recently, when it began to equalise, there was a peculiar disparity between the countries. The Swedes were suffering rates of asthma comparable to the worst affected nations of the world – Britain, New Zealand, Australia and the United States. While not unheard of in the other Baltic nations, it was markedly less common. Then the world underwent a seismic political shift, in 1989, and the map of Europe changed forever. The

Soviet Union collapsed, and the countries once subservient to its diktats were freed. Many countries altered their entire political, social, industrial and agricultural structures as a consequence. This was the moment when the trend for asthma and allergies in Latvia et al. began to change. Within a very few years, almost as many of the citizens of Tallinn were suffering from allergic conditions as their neighbours across the sea in Stockholm. Why should this be?

We know that environmental factors have an enormous impact on many diseases. Our diet in the West is supposed to have led to the epidemic of heart disease following the Second World War. Certain kinds of cancer have been associated with environmental factors since Victorian times: chimney sweeps were particularly prone to cancer of the scrotum; aniline dye workers to cancer of the bladder. Other lung diseases were known to be related to occupation: coal miners suffered from pneumoconiosis, while an unpleasant allergic condition known as farmer's lung affects a small proportion of people who work with hay. There are many other examples.

Inheritance has a great deal of effect on diseases, including the Quiet Killers. Susceptibility to particular infections, including TB, may be predicted by the presence or absence of certain genes. Certain ethnic groups – the Irish and the Somalis – are often said to be especially prone to catching TB. Other diseases, of course, also have a genetic element. Some cancers may be reliably predicted by genetic testing, so much so in the case of breast cancer that doctors may recommend the removal of healthy breasts. Although not directly inherited, a tendency to asthma may be observed in families.

Theories up to this point tended to try to explain asthma and hay fever as a combination of both factors: a genetically susceptible individual exposed to a suitable trigger would have a high chance of developing the disease. The trigger factors were believed at that time to be principally pollen, pollution, climate, and infections of the airways. What seemed to be happening in the ex-Soviet Baltic States required a subtler explanation. Pollen counts did not seem to have changed, nor had the climate, nor pollution. There did not seem to be any evidence of higher rates of infection among the population. The genetic make-up of the people had obviously not changed.

Various theories were tested. Many people felt that central heating might be responsible; the statistics did not support this hypothesis.

It may be worth taking a moment to consider the pathological processes that contribute to the condition called asthma; some of these features are shared with hay fever and other allergies. Asthma is caused by over-excitability of the tiny muscles that control the calibre of the airways. These muscles go into spasm, and air cannot easily pass through these constricted channels. The characteristic 'wheeze' of asthma is the audibly turbulent flow of air through the partly blocked passages. There is also inflammation of the airways, with leakage of fluids and white blood cells into the airways. The chemicals responsible for over-excitability of the airways and leakage of fluid are produced by white blood cells, or leukocytes. The white blood cells most implicated in the asthma response are called eosinophils and mast cells.

Asthma is, then, a disease caused by our own bodies. It is far from the only disease where this happens; among the Quiet Killers, the damage to the liver following infection with hepatitis B, and to the lungs with TB, is caused by our own immune systems. Both conditions may be usefully treated by drugs that modulate the immune response. Some doctors began to reflect on the other functions of the cells responsible for asthma, to see if there might be clues to causation of the illness.

Eosinophils, mast cells and related leukocytes also have actions in resisting invasion of the body from other infections. There are particular types of assault to which they are specifically adapted. These infections are the parasites – the tapeworms, cestodes and nematodes. They are also involved with the immune response to certain types of bacteria.

One feature of life in countries behind the old Iron Curtain could have been easily seen to have changed. The Soviet Union operated an agricultural system based on the collective farm. By western standards, these farms were poorly mechanised and required the involvement of large numbers of people to till the soil and harvest the crops. Further, many impoverished citizens in the political system which tended to suppress private enterprise would grow their own vegetables. Overall, most people would have had some connection to the soil. This changed forever with the fall of the Soviet Empire. Collective farms, which were inherently uncompetitive, collapsed in the new market economy. Many people were freed from the land; food was more frequently bought from supermarkets, often in the increasingly ubiquitous clingfilm packaging.

The 'hygiene hypothesis' therefore runs like this: we have evolved in constant exposure to many varieties of infection. Our immune responses reflect this; we have entire armies of leukocytes which are adapted to eradicating and controlling parasites. While we are exposed to these parasites, through regular contact with the soil, these white blood cells function smoothly. However, once our world becomes too 'clean', these cells lurk, unused, like massed ranks of cavalry waiting for the order to charge. When they encounter a substance that is superficially close enough to the structure of a parasite to activate them, they spring into action, releasing an abundance of chemicals that cause the airways to shut down, the nose to run, the skin to itch, and all the other manifestations of asthma, hay fever and allergies, up to and including death.

We may therefore have switched one Quiet Killer for another. The paradox is that asthma and allergies are probably more dangerous than the infections from which this branch of immunity protected us. Parasites like worms can and do kill, but asthma is an emerging killer in countries like the United States. Mortality doubled in that country between 1978 and 1989. Of course, improved hygiene protects us from other Quiet Killers like typhoid, cholera and dysentery. Thanks to improved public health, the risk of these illnesses is low anyway.

There is further convincing evidence to support the hygiene hypothesis. Severe asthma and allergy – particularly the increasingly common, sometimes fatal, nut allergies – are almost unheard of in places where tapeworm infections are common, such as Africa and India. In addition to the particular kinds of leukocytes which are shared between allergy and response to parasite infection, there is a specific immune protein implicated in both. Immune proteins are also known as immunoglobulins, and are classified by letters. This particular shared immunoglobulin is called Immunoglobulin E. It has two principal functions: to label parasite proteins as foreign and suitable for attack and destruction by white blood cells; and to signal to cells packed with histamine to release their contents. Histamine is one of the central chemicals responsible for the symptoms of asthma and allergy.

Proving that a 'dirty' lifestyle protects you from allergic disease is not easy. The challenge is plain: it is a culturally sensitive issue. How do you quantify 'dirtiness'? What is filth to one family is perfectly acceptable to another. For every person who believes that cleanliness is next to godliness, there is another who says you have to eat a bushel of dirt before you die.

There are some 'proxies' of lack of hygiene that have been used to provide circumstantial evidence. This theory states that it is more difficult to maintain hygiene in certain situations. The commonly quoted examples are: living in a large family with many brothers and sisters; going to a nursery; attending military camps and boarding schools; poverty; and overcrowding. People exposed to these are assumed to live less 'clean' lives; they can then be compared to people of identical age, sex and other characteristics to see which has the higher incidence of asthma and allergies. Some (but not all) of these studies have shown reasonably firm supporting evidence for the hygiene hypothesis.

There are obvious problems with the assumptions contained in such studies. First, it is by no means a certainty that each assumption is correct. Living in a large family may mean many different things – a wealthy family where every child has a single room is clearly different in this respect to the traditional Victorian caricature of a family of ten in a single bed. Such large families are, of course, far less common nowadays. Birth order will also play a part: the oldest child will clearly have a different experience to the youngest, who joins other siblings at the moment of birth. Some studies have taken this into account, and there does seem to be an effect whereby each successive child appears to have a slightly, but detectably, lower Immunoglobulin E.

However, the chief scientific difficulty with proxies is that they may accidentally represent something else that you hadn't considered. Suppose you were trying to devise a system for betting on racehorses. You notice that all the winners at a particular course had red blankets when seen in the paddock. You subsequently bet on every horse with a red blanket, and finish the day as a winner. The next time you visit a racecourse, you try the same strategy and lose your shirt. In this example, the proxy is the blanket, which of course belonged to a successful trainer or owner. This is a trivial example, but it is easy to be misled by using proxies. Suppose you designed a study that wanted to ask the question, is birth order important in subsequent development of asthma? You believed that a baby born to a family with two or more older siblings might be exposed to more bugs, and might therefore be protected. Your study confirms this. But what if the real cause of lower asthma in third and subsequent children were nothing to do with having brothers and sisters, but simply related to the age of the mother at the time of birth? Birth order would inevitably be a proxy for this, because with each pregnancy the mother inevitably becomes older.

There are, though, slightly more reliable markers of poor hygiene. Some diseases are principally transmitted by human faeces. One of these is hepatitis A, a disease of the liver that varies in symptoms from none at all to short-lived jaundice to, rarely, liver failure and death. Evidence of hepatitis A infection may be considered a sound proxy for poor hygiene, on the principle that even the most slovenly domestic arrangements tend to avoid contact with human faeces. The added advantage of using this as a marker is that previous infection may be detected by a simple blood test, which is either positive or negative, and remains so for life. An Italian scientist called Matricardi devised a series of elegant experiments to test the theory that people who had been exposed to more germs in childhood, as suggested by a positive test for hepatitis A, would have less of the particular proteins associated with asthma in their blood. This protein Immunoglobulin is called 'aeroallergen specific IgE'. Matricardi studied a group of military recruits. His hypothesis was confirmed – the recruits that tested positive for hepatitis A had aeroallergen specific IgE concentrations half that of the negative recruits. Hepatitis A infection is, however, also associated with large family size and poverty. It was important to check that these factors were not responsible for the findings. It is possible to test such a hypothesis statistically; in this case, it was not so. Being exposed to hepatitis A – and therefore, other bugs – seemed to provide evidence of protection against asthma, irrespective of the size of your family or their poverty. This study has been repeated in Aberdeen, Scotland, with the same conclusion. Matricardi has repeated his experiments on non-military individuals in the community, with the same outcome. He has also tested his theory against other bugs that are spread by the same route, *Toxoplasma gondii* and *Helicobacter pylori*. The results were the same.

These experiments, although very suggestive, do not answer a very important question. Is the hepatitis A virus actually directly responsible for the effect, by interacting with the immune system, or is it just a 'proxy' for exposure to other germs? Matricardi believes the second of these hypotheses. He believes that our immune systems are 'primed' during a critical period in our lives, during which exposure to infections is 'expected' by our white blood cells exactly like the example of BCG discssed below. Other scientists have noted that people leading what may be called a 'traditional lifestyle' – life in the open, in the fields, with multiple successive infections – have far lower incidence of atopy, suggesting that we need exposure to lots of germs, not just hepatitis A. This is more than just an academic point. As Matricardi says, 'If we knew how high microbial turnover "educates" our immune system, perhaps we could learn to mimic its action without giving up our hygienic lifestyle.' In other words, simply adopting a 'dirty' lifestyle is too risky, although probably very appealing to many young children. If exposure to many different kinds of germs is required – as seems somehow plausible, given the *toxoplasma* and *helicobacter* data – then a narrowly directed vaccine would not work. However, if you knew for certain that some part of the hepatitis A virus interacted with your immune system to protect you from asthma and atopy, you might be able to isolate that single viral constituent and use it as a vaccine for allergy. Using just that viral constituent, without the rest of the virus, would avoid the risk of developing hepatitis, which has a mortality of about 1 per cent.

There is a further caveat. Some germs may have far more unwelcome consequences. *Helicobacter pylori* is a bacterium transmitted by the faecal route. As indicated above, it has been shown in one study to be associated with a reduction in blood levels of proteins associated with asthma. *Helicobacter* is not harmless, however; it is now widely accepted as the cause of stomach ulcers and even cancers. One very small study has also connected it to Sudden Infant Death Syndrome. This is the difficulty in harnessing the hygiene hypothesis to our benefit. Avoiding the Quiet Killers may not be entirely wholesome; embracing them is dangerous too.

There is more. It may not just be parasites like tapeworms that modulate our response to the environment. Other life forms, including bacteria, do the same thing. For a long time, doctors were baffled by conflicting and inconsistent results with vaccination for one of the most dangerous of the Quiet Killers – TB. The vaccine is called BCG, or Bacille Calmette–Guérin, after its inventors. BCG is a modified version of a bacterium related to TB, *Mycobacterium bovis*. As its name suggests, this organism causes TB in cattle, only very rarely doing so in humans. As we discussed in Chapter Three, BCG vaccine seemed to work in some countries but not in others such as Burma.

How could you explain this conundrum? One by one, the following perfectly reasonable hypotheses have been discounted. There was enough difference between batches of vaccine to affect the outcome. There are genetic differences between peoples and races which cause them to respond to vaccines differently in different countries. The information was collected in different ways in different countries. None of these really resolved the paradox.

There is, however, a hypothesis which fits the facts most neatly. *Mycobacterium tuberculosis* has cousins, and they are everywhere. They belong to a group known to scientists as the 'acid-fast bacilli', so called because the stains used to detect them are not bleached out by acids. There are at least fifty mycobacterial species. Only a very small fraction of this number cause disease, the leprosy bacterium being one of them. A few others will cause illness under rare and peculiar conditions. *Mycobacterium marinum*, for instance, causes a skin eruption called 'Fish Fancier's Finger' in keepers of tropical fish who clean their own tanks with ungloved hands. Some mycobacteria, such as *Mycobacterium chelonei* and *Mycobacterium avium*, are only able to cause illness in people with damaged lungs and immunity caused by rare inherited defects or AIDS. *Mycobacterium scrofulaceum* causes swelling of the lymph nodes in susceptible people; this is the ancient condition of scrofula, or the 'King's Evil'. Lymph glands, usually in the neck, swell up and may even ulcerate. Edward the Confessor was supposedly able to cure this disease by simple touch. You will have encountered these cousins of the Captain of the Men of Death, but almost certainly without realising it. They are everywhere: in tap water, in food, even in hospital sterilising systems. Their resistance to acid and alcohol allows them to shrug off many chemical means of decontamination. Your immune system, however, will have triumphed in the encounter and contained the assault. However, like an army fraternising with the enemy, that immune system will have been altered.

What appears to happen is that each brush with these bacteria primes the immune cells in a directed and irreversible manner. According to this hypothesis, the key to the outcome is precisely which of these common organisms you encounter first. Some will skew your immunity down a path that will protect you from subsequent infection with TB. Others will have the opposite effect, rendering you more likely to develop disease. There are two further possible consequences of this second, less favourable outcome. One is that you may be more likely to develop asthma and allergies. Indeed, the disease of TB has much in common with an exaggerated allergic reaction. The second is that further inoculation with other mycobacteria such as the BCG vaccine will not protect you from infection; in fact, it may even make you more susceptible. That is the best explanation to date of the Burmese conundrum – in Burma, the commonly encountered environmental mycobacteria are the sort that render the Burmese more, not less, susceptible to TB. In Britain, where BCG appears to confer some protection, we are exposed to a different set of environmental mycobacteria.

There is a little more circumstantial, and paradoxical, evidence to support the hypothesis. In western countries, children are frequently – rightly or wrongly – given antibiotics for minor infections. One convincing study has shown that children given antibiotics in the early years of life are far more likely to develop asthma and allergies in later years. Certain antibiotics – notably, erythromycin – may be more prone to provoking this response. Such medications are lethal to many mycobacteria. Ironically, they are often prescribed where there is anxiety about inducing a penicillin allergy.

Overall, there is accumulating and convincing evidence to suggest that we may need some exposure to bugs and dirt to keep our immune systems busy and out of mischief. As has been said, atopy and infection may be two sides of the same coin – the appropriate response to some kinds of infection is a specialised form of 'allergy'. Nonetheless, all of this remains simply hypothetical at present. Some doctors have nevertheless sought to take it further. Joel Weinstock of the University of Iowa has treated a group of patients with bowel disorders, such as Crohn's disease and ulcerative colitis, by deliberately infecting them with a tapeworm called *Trichuris suis*, with some success. A team in Britain, led by Professors John Stanford and Graham Rook, has been attempting to treat a range of conditions using naturally occurring TB-like mycobacteria.

The hygiene hypothesis is an attractive one, for many reasons. It has some rational scientific basis, which I have partly explained above. It fits many of the facts quite neatly. But, more than this, it strikes a chord with a society which has become wary of 'progress', which looks back wistfully to a supposedly happier time, where the kind of advice handed out by grizzled matriarchs to get outdoors and eat your bushel of dirt was heeded above that of scientists. The French even have a term for this: '*nostalgie de la boue*'. However, although passing the test of logical plausibility is important, the other considerations should make us regard the hypothesis with more suspicion rather than less, because they tend to cloud the scientific judgement. We should therefore conclude that the jury is still out. Keep washing your hands.

Some scientists believe that any biological hypothesis that cannot be explained within the context of Darwinian evolution is flawed and should be automatically rejected. The hygiene hypothesis certainly appears to fulfil those criteria. We evolved alongside the Quiet Killers. It isn't surprising that our immunity is designed to withstand assault from a variety of infectious challenges. Only the most recent generations have lived in our relatively sterile, air-conditioned, centrally heated environment. Mechanisation post Industrial Revolution has drastically reduced the proportion of people habitually exposed to the soil. A hypothesis which postulates that for the first time whole branches of our immune systems are surplus to requirements clearly meets our evolutionary shibboleth. However, there is plenty of other evidence that infection and human evolution have operated hand-in-hand.

In fact, we may owe both our whole existence and our mortality to the Quiet Killers. This is one of the most bizarre and paradoxical of all the infections. It is not one that preys on and sustains humans alone, but all higher organisms. It is the most chronic, in the sense of prolonged, infection of all time. This infection happened to us about two billion years ago. It seems reasonable to classify it as a Quiet Killer, because it is still killing us. Without this infection, we would never have emerged from the primordial ooze; because of it, our allotted span is limited, our faculties fail after a certain time, we age, we wither and we die. Shakespeare's sonnet on Time could have been written about this infection, because it 'doth transfix the flourish set on youth, / And delves the parallels in beauty's brow [. . .] And yet to times in hope my verse shall stand, / Praising thy worth, despite his cruel hand.'

Life, according to one system of classification, can be divided into two major groups. One is called the prokaryotes, the other eukaryotes. Humans belong to the second category, the eukaryotes. There are many differences between the two, but for the sake of this discussion we will concentrate on just one. Within almost all cells of eukaryotes, there is a separate structure, the nucleus, separated from the rest of the contents of the cell by a membrane. The delicate, vulnerable DNA of the genes is enveloped in this nucleus. Prokaryotes lack this nucleus; all of their functions occur jumbled up together in the rich soup inside the cell called the cytoplasm. The greater majority of the Quiet Killers are prokaryotes; certainly, all bacteria fall into this category. The nucleus in eukaryotes has many functions within its delicate contents. It is surrounded by a membrane which protects it from very dangerous structures lodged in its cytoplasm. These structures are called mitochondria, and very odd things they are too. It is something of a mystery as to why or how they got there. One thing we are absolutely certain about, though – they arose as bacteria, and infected us, and got stuck there.

We know that mitochondria arose in bacteria for several very convincing reasons: they look like bacteria; they behave like bacteria; they are made of bacterial proteins and DNA; and they reproduce like bacteria. New mitochondria arise only by the division of existing mitochondria; that is, they reproduce asexually, like bacteria and unlike humans. If they are lost or damaged, the cell cannot replace them, unlike other human cell structures. Mitochondria always remain separate entities within the cell, unlike other human cell compartments which are constantly fusing with one another – sending off and absorbing little packages in bubbles, and generally interacting inside the cell. Mitochondria have their own DNA and machinery for making proteins, which are of bacterial type and distinct from that of humans. If you compare the DNA and proteins of mitochondria with other bacteria in the evolutionary tree, they are clearly bacteria themselves. They belong to a group called the Alphaproteobacteria. Their closest living relatives are the purple sulphur bacteria and the *Rickettsiae*. This latter group is particularly tantalising. *Rickettsiae* are a group of organisms that will be discussed elsewhere; they are responsible for diseases like typhus. One of their key features is that they are deficient in a cell wall and can only cause infection by parasitically invading the contents of another cell.

There are other examples of cells becoming permanently infected by bacteria, and with similarly unpredictable consequences. Some strains of amoebae can be infected experimentally with bacteria in the laboratory. As with most species, some of the amoebae resist infection; some die; and some survive, but are left with persistent infection. Initially, the infection slows the amoebae down – they are less active and reproduce more slowly. Gradually, however, they regain their vigour. Now here's the amazing part: if these recovered amoebae are treated with antibiotics to kill the bacteria, the amoebae die too. In other words, the amoebae have somehow become dependent on the invading bacteria.

If you ask a cell biologist why eukaryotes have mitochondria, they will usually answer, 'to provide energy'. This is true – up to a point. Mitochondria are like little furnaces, churning out energy in a form that cells can use. However, bacteria that lack mitochondria are perfectly capable of producing their own energy. Why eukaryotes need mitochondria is unclear. What does seem true is that obtaining mitochondria allows organisms to develop a level of structural complexity that is impossible without them; this will be explained in slightly more detail below.

Having mitochondria – and each eukaryotic cell has many – is far from wholly beneficial, and this is why I have included them among our Quiet Killers. First, they produce toxic waste products. Imperfectly combusted oxygen molecules are highly poisonous to cells. They are known as free radicals, or 'Reactive Oxygen Species'. About 90 per cent of such radicals produced within a cell are generated from mitochondria. Such toxic waste products are largely responsible for the fact that we age. The mitochondria themselves are particularly vulnerable to this damage; by the age of 65, about half of our mitochondria have stopped working properly. DNA from mitochondria is more susceptible to mutation than human DNA; these little parasites actually age faster than we do.

There is a convincing hypothesis to explain all of this rather dense information. About two billion years ago, a primitive organism was attacked by another, either a purple sulphur bacterium or a *Rickettsia*. Once the attacking bacterium had invaded the cell, instead of destroying it, it discovered a niche in which it could survive. Deficient in cell wall, it liked the protected environment of the cytoplasm in which it found itself. The invaded cell discovered, abruptly, that it had acquired a whole new set of genes and a source of energy, bypassing several million years of necessary evolution to reach the same stage. This allowed it to evolve at a far higher rate than other competing organisms. It was able to concentrate on other functions than the simple daily scramble for energy; this task had been sub-contracted out to the mitochondria. There was a price to pay, however. The new lodger had a rather poisonous smoking habit, which caused both landlord and tenant to age faster than they otherwise would. We are the direct descendants of this little housing cooperative, and we have not escaped the same drawback. The presence of this Quiet Killer in our cells has been so useful to us that we have tolerated its evil habits for too long to evict it. This process is called symbiogenesis.

You may well reasonably argue at this point that it is all very well for our imaginary primitive beast to have acquired this parasite, but surely when it reproduced its offspring would lose it? Just because mother or father was infected, surely the child would be spared unless re-infected. The answer is, not so. There are many examples of parasitic infections being transmitted from mother to offspring; this is known as transovarial infection and is commonplace. But this phenomenon provides another key to the nature of ageing and mitochondrial invasion. Mitochondria reproduce asexually. In other words, each successive generation cannot acquire new genes. Thus, they are almost incapable of evolving to protect themselves. This makes them more susceptible to irreversible decay and ageing. We are, therefore, at the mercy of these fragile and ancient life forms, and they determine our life-span.

In a sense, all life is either bacteria or descends from bacteria: life *is* bacteria. A biologist called Lynn Margulis proposes that our bodies are amalgams of several different strains of them; this is called endosymbiosis, and it means that bacteria are responsible for the creation of all complex forms of life. The merger of organisms referred to above is also known to have happened many times in biological history, and is even responsible for the Origin of Species. All life began with viruses and bacteria. Bacteria merged to form more complex, but still single-celled, algae and amoebae. These merged again to form more complex organisms; fungi, plants and animals.

Life on Earth is still dominated by bacteria. In terms of biomass, they easily form the greater majority of life. They maintain the conditions for life on the planet. The air we breathe, the stuff we are made from – all relies on these tiny organisms. Rather like the white mice in *The Hitchhiker's Guide to the Galaxy*, you could almost argue that the bacteria are really in charge. Bodies are suitable food sources for bacteria. Bacteria have merged into complex structures that provide them with effective sources of nutrients; that includes us. We are being 'farmed' by the Quiet Killers.

The greater environment is controlled mostly by bacteria; it is, in a sense, 'their' environment, not ours. They even determine some of the geology of our planet. Certain mineral deposits have been shaped by the work of bacteria over millions of years, or by reaction with the waste gas of bacteria. We have evolved to live in their effluent which maintains a balance of chemicals in the air that we can breathe. All life relies on them. We do not live in the Age of Man; we live in the Age of Bacteria.

As far as the Quiet Killers are concerned, our relatively recent more sophisticated understanding of these life forms has enabled us to identify, evade and combat the most obviously dangerous candidates. Despite the emergence of resistance, there are very few disease-causing types which are untreatable. It is important to understand, though, that the classification of a bacterium as disease-causing may be highly situation-specific, and that our immersion in them in general has both positive and negative possibilities. The ability of any bacterium to become a killer may be entirely circumstantial.

Most people are aware that their intestines are colonised with bacteria. We dismiss this as a commonplace, without noting a number of astonishing features of this remarkable tenancy. Few of us appreciate the sheer scale of the accommodation provided. There are more individual cells of bacteria in our intestines than there are individual cells in our bodies. Nor are bacteria confined to our guts. Almost every surface is colonised with germs of one sort or another, including our eyes. Here, then, is one paradox, which I shall call the near-miss. Every time you or I walk along a road busy with traffic, we are only feet, inches sometimes, away from disaster. A single false step along the pavement and we could be under a lorry. Without really thinking about it, we know that if we keep our course without stumbling we are safe. So it is with the Quiet Killers. The fact that they live on our skins or in our guts without doing damage does not mean that they are harmless. They are like juggernauts swinging by us at 80 miles per hour, but as long as we don't trip under their wheels we are fine. One of the most numerous in our intestines is called *Escherichia coli*. For the most part, we live harmoniously with this organism. However, it is perfectly capable of becoming a killer. Disease-causing variants may infect the intestine. Even the 'harmless' variant may kill or cause severe disease if it contaminates a wound or a site that should be sterile, for example the bladder. Many of the most dangerous infections are caused by bacteria that otherwise live harmlessly on our skins or in our throats. *Neisseria meningitidis* can cause meningococcal meningitis, which is 100 per cent fatal if untreated. It happily lives in the throat of 15 per cent of normal people. Another common organism found in the throat is *Streptococcus pneumoniae*, the cause of the commonest sort of pneumonia – the sort suffered by Marianne Dashwood in Jane Austen's *Sense and Sensibility* – has a 30 per cent mortality if untreated. It is found in the throats of 10 per cent of otherwise healthy people. Even MRSA, chief among our current bogeymen, can live harmlessly on our skins. The reasons that these guests occasionally bite the hand that feeds them are discussed elsewhere.

The presence of some of these bacteria is often transient. You will not be surprised to learn, though, given the complexity of the interactions between microbes and man, that much of it is not pure chance. First, we make use of them. Bacteria and yeasts in our intestine are vital to digestion. Particularly in the large intestine, they digest carbohydrates, proteins and lipids that have arrived in unaltered form from the small intestine. This is more important in ruminants; nonetheless, humans also rely on them to break down vegetable matter. Next, the bacteria that colonise us are not like passive colonies in a petri dish. They interact with each other; they talk to each other; and, more astonishingly, they talk to us and we talk to them, requesting and being granted permission to remain where they are. They have other functions, though, which may startle you: they help our sex drive, and they make women beautiful.

Human sexual activity relies on a type of steroid. Both testosterone and oestrogen are sex steroids and are derived from a common source, called deoxycholic acid. Bacteria in the intestine convert cholic acid, which is released from the liver through the bile duct into the gut, to deoxycholic acid. Without deoxycholic acid, there can be no testosterone and no oestrogen. Testosterone is responsible for libido in both the male and the female. Oestrogen has been shown in some studies to be responsible for the sexual attractiveness of females. In other words, people rely on the contents of their colon to attract one another. This is a slightly facetious simplification. Other human tissues are capable of metabolising sex steroids. But the significance of the action of these bacteria is demonstrated by the fact that antibiotics that disturb the balance of germs in the small intestine can lead to unwanted pregnancy. They do so by killing the bacteria that have been metabolising oestrogen in the contraceptive pill.

Bacteria also provide us with some protection from their more dangerous cousins. The best way to obtain a weed-free lawn is to encourage a dense crop of particular mixed grass varieties that compete successfully against weeds for light, water and nutrients. Once this is achieved, then the lawn requires far less maintenance, and ugly mosses and weeds find it much harder to establish themselves. So it is with the colonising bacteria of our skin and intestines. The optimum is a garden of mixed organisms that are able to live happily with us, consuming organic matter and oils produced on our skin surfaces. Their physical presence, as well as the fact that bacteria can actually poison other species, prevents colonisation by other bugs that can produce dangerous toxins and chemicals. The commonest organism on our skin is known as

Staphylococcus epidermidis, although this has many sub-types, rather like lawn grass. This bacterium is the conscientious objector of the world of *Staphylococci*. It produces very few toxins that damage humans, and is a near-perfect skin organism for us.

Staphylococcus epidermidis is not universally benign, and can revert to Quiet Killer status. As in my near-miss example above, it can behave like a juggernaut if we slip under its wheels. One of the reasons the bacterium colonises our skins so successfully is that it has sophisticated methods of attaching tightly to many sorts of surfaces. If the surface happens to be an artificial hip joint or heart valve, or the intravenous drip of a sick baby, then *S. epidermidis* can turn nasty.

Suppose the weeds on a lawn begin to get out of hand. The lawn might best be treated with weedkiller. This may, of course, be beneficial. However, sometimes it may cause bare patches to appear, either where weeds and moss have died, or, sometimes, where patches of grass die, particularly if the dose is accidentally miscalculated. The analogy here is, obviously, treatment with antibiotics. It is sadly impossible at present to create 'designer' antibiotics that kill only bacteria that are causing disease. All bacteria that are susceptible to the agent used will be killed. This will leave gaps in the lawn, which can be replaced by less welcome guests. The classical example of this is thrush of the mouth or vagina; this is caused by the yeast *Candida albicans*, which replaces the usual healthy flora, with painful consequences. More seriously, a bacterium called *Clostridium difficile* may spill over into these bare patches in the intestine. This bacterium produces very dangerous poisons that can cause a range of symptoms, from nothing at all through severe diarrhoea to massive swelling and fatal rupture of the colon.

You may think this lawn analogy contrived and far-fetched. However, the analogy is closer than you might think. To check the health of a lawn, it needs to be inspected to be certain that the species growing there are the desirable ones. If this is not the case, there will be necessary remedies. Our bodies do exactly the same with bacteria. They garden, farm, till and cultivate them. Surface colonisation is an inexact description of the location of bacteria on our skins and in our guts. They are attached very intimately to our cells, some of whose function is to inspect them and ensure they are safe – exactly like a gardener inspecting a lawn. If they are the wrong ones, in health they are removed by the equivalent of taking a trowel to them – a process known as phagocytosis, where the bacteria are enveloped and destroyed. But more than this, our skins, tears and secretions are also capable of producing selective weedkillers. These are the cationic anti-microbial peptides. For example, your skin produces a chemical called dermcidin. Many of them are species-specific; that is, they aim to leave the welcome guests on your body while killing the more dangerous ones. Actually, dermcidin is better than weedkiller, because it signals to alert the immune responses to possible attack. We will meet it again; it has not escaped the surveillance of scientists.

*   *   *

The Quiet Killers may have been responsible for our evolution in a slightly deeper, more philosophical way. We will call this the Red Queen hypothesis, after the character in Lewis Carroll's *Alice in Wonderland*. The Red Queen, you will remember, had to run faster and faster in order to stay in the same place. Imagine a species of animal that has a very rudimentary and basic immune system. This animal is primitive, but plentiful. Suppose that animal meets, for the first time, an infection. The majority of the infected animals will die; however, some may survive. The survivors will be those whose immune system, by chance, has a mutation which makes it slightly more effective than the others. With luck, that mutation will be passed on to the progeny of the surviving animal. Suppose this process is repeated on multiple occasions with fresh infections. It is not hard to see that a species of greater complexity and sophistication will arise. Suppose that one of the adaptations which emerges as particularly successful in resisting infection is one that is able to respond very rapidly to an infectious challenge. It does so by triggering fast electrical impulses. These electrical impulses might simply cause infection-fighting chemicals to be instantly released from a store, instead of employing the far slower process of building them from scratch. This is very basic and primitive physiology. Nonetheless, we have the rudiments of the *sine qua non* of human existence and consciousness – a nervous system. Without the challenge of the infection, the animal would not have had to develop anything as complex as this; the Red Queen would not even have had to get out of bed, let alone break into a trot.

There are indubitably infections that are good for us, but as we have seen we walk a tightrope. In the face of the threat from the Quiet Killers, all of our body systems have evolved to respond to infection. They do so in a complex and coordinated way. The consequence is that systems that you might not expect to be involved with fighting infection – the endocrine system, for example – probably evolved more rapidly and to a higher degree of sophistication than they would have accomplished without that challenge. In other words, without the Quiet Killers, we would not be who we are; and you could speculate that consciousness might never have evolved. There are those who believe that human consciousness arose due to a viral infection; such claims are so speculative as to be almost science fiction and I do not propose to discuss them further.

Much of what has been discussed in this chapter concerning infections that are good for us, although fascinating and credible, remains speculative and theoretical. The evidence is compelling, yet none of it is quite proven – and how could you conclusively prove something, such as the endosymbiosis theory, that supposedly happened about two billion years ago? However, there is one quirky infection that has shown promise as one that really can save lives; and an oddity it is, too. Some patients with HIV and AIDS have been carefully studied in groups for many years; the object being to try to identify factors that might prolong or reduce survival. One such group is the American Multicenter AIDS Cohort, a large group of gay men with AIDS who have been followed since 1984. In 2004, a startling discovery was made about men in this group. Some of them had developed a second viral infection. The virus in question is closely related to deadly hepatitis C, and when it was first discovered it was presumed that it would cause similar types of illness. It is known as GB Virus-C, after the initials of the virologist who first described it.

When it became clear that GBV-C did not seem to cause disease, many scientists lost interest in it. Those that continued to monitor its effects were rewarded with a remarkable discovery: after six years of infection with GBV-C, twice as many men survived as those who were uninfected. In other words, something about this virus seemed to combat AIDS. No other virus has ever been shown to do this. Whether or not this peculiarity will translate into useful medical treatment remains to be seen. Nonetheless, once again it illustrates the astounding capacity of infectious agents to defy our preconceptions.

Before we move on to infections that are definitely not good for us – indeed those that might kill us all – I will end on a tantalising note about the nature of who and what we are. When the human genome, that essential blueprint within every one of us, was unravelled, something distinctly odd emerged. Patterns of genes were discerned that seemed to arise from somewhere else, somewhere not human. They are termed 'mobile genetic elements'. They come predominantly from viruses, but also bacteria. We know that they are not human because of the products the genes encode. In a sense, this is not surprising – all organisms are susceptible to viruses, which by their nature incorporate into the DNA of the host. Some are viruses very similar to HIV, called human endogenous retroviruses (HERVs). We could dismiss their presence, apart from two facts. One is that we actually use these mobile genetic elements – for example, the protein syncitin is a HERV product vital for successful pregnancy. What is even more amazing is the sheer number of them. Almost half of our DNA derives from viruses and bacteria. We are made of the Quiet Killers.

SEVEN

Annihilators and Destroyers
Diseases that could kill us all

In previous chapters, we have looked at diseases that could have or have already killed millions. Plague, TB, influenza, smallpox, malaria – all have a butcher's bill extending to many millions of lives. Nevertheless, the human race soldiers on. If we trouble ourselves over the possible extinction of our species, our anxieties lie in the wanton misuse of our natural resources, climate change, asteroid collision or, until recently (and now possibly again), global nuclear war. The Quiet Killers have been erased from our list of absolute threats to our existence. Is that reasonable? Is there such a thing as an infection that could kill every single one of us?

We have seen elsewhere the consequences of infections that have been introduced to previously unexposed populations – the havoc wrought by measles among Pacific Islanders, for instance, and the disease-assisted triumph of conquistadores over the Aztecs. These infections were catastrophic and caused the collapse of sophisticated and powerful civilisations. They did not, however, wipe out everyone infected. There are reasons for this.

First, the infection was transmitted from Europeans in whom measles was endemic. The term endemic requires more careful definition for the purposes of this discussion. It means that the illness has reached a state of equilibrium within a population: immunity and disease have reached a balance. People still fall ill from the disease, and some may even die, but there are many more who contract low-grade, trivial infections that simply result in long-term immunity. For this state of equilibrium to occur without vaccination, several things must happen. First, the population affected must have a sufficiently adaptable immune system to

134

develop effective antibodies to the infection. Next, the virus must continue to circulate naturally in order to generate immunity by acquired infection. Finally, if the original infection had a high epidemic mortality, the virus must change and attenuate its virulence. Thus alastrim is a modified, low-virulence form of smallpox; in endemic populations, measles is usually a mild condition. Even with the Pacific Islanders and the Aztecs, the chances are that some of the population would be infected with the virus of lower virulence. In time even the virulent form would mutate to the attenuated. Furthermore, measles is not an absolutely unique virus. It belongs to a group of related viruses, the paramyxoviruses, which include canine distemper. Most people will have been exposed to paramyxoviruses. There will, therefore, be some primitive priming of the immune system to similar infections. However weak, this will provide sufficient protection to allow survival of some of the population.

In order to provide a threat to the whole of humankind, two conditions must therefore be met by our putative Quiet Killer. First, it must not only be entirely unencountered by humans, but it must have no close relatives either. Of course, there would have to be other characteristics – readily transmitted, fatal, not susceptible to any available drugs – but these two are the chief ones. Where could such a new infection arise? The majority of 'new' diseases (discussed in Chapter Ten) have arisen from wild, farmed or domestic animals. Even HIV is now believed to have arisen by this route, through the butchering of wild apes; the virus, which belongs to the retrovirus family, has relatives in cat, seal and even human infections. The likelihood of our encountering entirely new infections by animal encounter is therefore small. There really is 'nothing new under the sun'.

What about 'over the sun'? There was anxiety at one time about the introduction of viruses from space; HIV was briefly postulated to have arrived via a meteorite. The *Jurassic Park* author Michael Crichton, himself a doctor, dealt with such a hypothesis in his first novel, *The Andromeda Strain*. Published in 1971, it concerns the US Army's 'Scoop' satellite programme which attempts to collect space pathogens for use in biological warfare. A couple of years later, Scoop VII crashes in Arizona. A virus with a prodigious capacity for mutation is released, which proceeds to wreak havoc.

Without wishing to be excessively categorical, a space-bound route is as about as unlikely as the reconstructed dinosaurs of *Jurassic Park*. Viruses are not robust when separated from their host cells. They can survive on inanimate objects – SARS (Severe Auto Respiratory Syndrome; see below) was probably initially spread on infected elevator buttons – but the conditions of ultra-violet radiation in space and the extreme heat of entry into Earth's atmosphere make viral survival in meteorites unlikely, if not impossible. Nor is survival on the suit of a returning astronaut really likely, or borne out by events from real extra-terrestrial travel.

A more plausible source for an entirely new infection is someone fiddling about in a laboratory somewhere and coming up with something horrible, accidentally or otherwise. It is not only plant material that may be genetically modified. Viruses are, by their nature, highly suitable for snipping, trimming, adding to or extending. Viruses are basically packets of genetic information contained in an envelope of varying degrees of sophistication. Some, but not all, contain enzymes that trigger their own replication when they infect a cell. Some force the host to produce the necessary enzymes for them. The function of some of these enzymes may be to act as splicers – they recognise specific gene sequences and snip them out, then re-insert them elsewhere. This is how viruses work, by inserting their genetic information into a suitable victim's genes. If the correct target gene sequence for splicing is present, the enzyme will work on any gene whether or not it belongs to the original virus. It is not a major leap from understanding this information to creating an entirely new virus, one that mankind has never encountered before. What would happen then? We know the answer to this. We know it from the animal kingdom, from rabbits.

The expression 'breeding like rabbits' is a just one. Unlike most mammals, the female rabbit *Oryctolagus cuniculus* produces fertile eggs as a consequence of mating. Rabbits are not native to many of the countries in which they are now found. They were artificially introduced to Britain, for example, from the Mediterranean and from North Africa as a crop – for fur and food – about 900 years ago. Like so many farmed imported species, they escaped from captivity and rapidly established feral populations numbering many millions. They were introduced to Australia in 1759 by Thomas Austin, for sport hunting. Almost all of the rabbits in Australia are descendants of his twenty-four original rabbits. The presence of these imported animals mattered little for many years, until farming practices changed during the mid-nineteenth century. By the early twentieth century, the rabbits were reproducing with astonishing success, and began to be perceived as a pest. Efforts by farmers to eradicate them were largely unsuccessful, until they began to experiment with viruses.

Dr P.F. Armand-Delille was a retired physician who lived in a rabbit-infested estate at Maillebois in northern France near Paris. In mid-1952, this irritable medic could bear the rabbits no longer and decided to take action. He knew of highly successful experiments to control rabbit populations in Australia during the previous year. In those days, such biological equipment could be obtained relatively easily, and so he managed to obtain some of the responsible material. He inoculated two wild rabbits. The agent was, of course, myxomatosis.

In autumn 1953, the disease arrived in Britain at the town of Edenbridge in Kent. Panicked Ministry of Agriculture officials tried to contain it. This was doomed to failure by the nature of the infection and the nature of the rabbit. The disease is partly transmitted between animals by mosquitoes and the rabbit flea; but some farmers, seeing an opportunity to eradicate a creature long detested as a menace to agriculture and woodland, spread the disease deliberately. Such actions were criminalised by the Pests Act of 1954, although hardly anyone was actually prosecuted. Within a few years, 99 per cent of Britain's rabbits were dead.

Myxomatosis is a naturally occurring illness of wild rabbits of a slightly different species, *Sylvilagus brasiliensis*. This strain is common in South America, including Uruguay. In Montevideo in 1896, it was noticed that, in contrast to the wild local strain, the recently imported European rabbit had a marked susceptibility to this infection. The wild rabbits suffered mild and transient symptoms when exposed, but just a whiff of the virus and *Oryctolagus cuniculus* dropped dead. By 1919, the disease had been identified as a potential solution to the persistent problem of rabbits as agricultural pests. It was tested in Britain and Australia, finally being released to catastrophic effect (for the rabbits) in Australia in 1950–1. It seemed a natural and superbly efficient pest eradicator, which would exterminate an unwelcome and introduced species. Fortuitously, it did not seem to jump the species barrier to other livestock or to humans. I say fortuitously deliberately; the possibility of humans contracting myxomatosis was barely considered in 1951 when it was released into Australia. There were other unexpected consequences in Europe, though – the buzzard population in particular suffered a serious setback; grass on downlands quickly became long since there were fewer rabbits; and attacks by foxes on hen roosts and game became more frequent.

The current British rabbit population is about half of what it was prior to 1953 when the virus arrived in Kent; current estimates put the figure at 30 million. The Australian rabbit population has similarly recovered. How can this be? Myxomatosis killed nearly all the rabbits, who had no immunity to this virus. Surely it should have killed them all? Would a similar infection kill all of us?

To understand what happened to the disease, and gain insight into how a similar outbreak might develop in a human population, it is necessary to look at the virus and its life cycle in a little more detail. Myxomatosis is a member of the Poxvirus family, related to smallpox and Jenner's *vaccinia* virus. It is about 280 nanometres (billionths of a metre) in length, which is actually quite large by viral standards. It is principally transmitted between animals by insects, including fleas and mosquitoes. The fleas may live on in the warren of a wiped-out colony and re-infect the next rabbit who tries to live there. The illness may also be spread by direct contact with diseased tissues. However, the most successful outbreaks of myxomatosis with the highest mortality occurred during the summer months, when the main vector was the mosquito.

Several things changed to save the European rabbit. First, the virus became a victim of its own success. In order to persist and survive, an infection that kills all its possible victims is going to be onto a loser since it will not be able to survive itself. It is like a king who imprisons everyone who fails to pay his excessive taxes – eventually, he will run out of citizens to tax, and even run out of jailers. In the early years of an outbreak, where the rate of spread of the disease is limited by geography, this may not matter. Ultimately, however, the virus will die out with the susceptible victims. There are several possible means for the virus to escape this fate. It can infect a different species to form a separate reservoir. This was not an option for myxomatosis, as there was no susceptible animal in Europe or Australia available for it to infect. It can mutate into a less virulent form; ideally, one that can lie dormant for long periods and occasionally wake up to re-infect. Finally, its victim can change to become more resistant to the infection. All viruses mutate, at a greater rate than most other life forms. It is an inevitable rule of evolution that a mutation which tends to enhance the survival of an organism will persist. Such a mutation in a highly fatal infection would therefore seem to be inevitable. It seems that such a mutation has occurred: myxomatosis in Australia now kills only about 40 per cent of infected rabbits.

A virus that kills 99 per cent of rabbits will nevertheless leave a lot of rabbits if there were a lot to start with. To be exact, 600,000 in the UK, if our initial figure of 60 million was correct. There may be several features of those surviving rabbits which made their escape more likely. If they were less active in the summer months, for instance, they might have escaped the mosquitoes. If they had tended to be less sociable, and less likely to spend time in the burrows than their cousins, they might have escaped both infection by direct contact and infection by fleas within the warren. In a state where the rabbits were uninfected, these behavioural traits might actually be disadvantageous to the rabbits – unsociable, inactive rabbits are presumably less likely to reproduce. Thus, a population which survives might actually be less reproductively successful than the original population. This is borne out by the figures: despite the legendary mating capacity of the rabbit, in fifty years the British population has only returned to about half of its previous number. There is a further important point to be made here: in order for the rabbit population to survive by adaptation, the behaviour is more likely to be genetically determined; otherwise, the characteristics cannot be passed on to the offspring and the virus can re-infect. It is possible, of course, that the rabbits are teaching their offspring to behave differently. A hard-wired, genetic adaptation is more likely to be successful; behavioural traits are more likely to revert.

Why haven't the rabbits just evolved immunity to the virus? Presumably, if there are 60 million to start with then some must, accidentally, have an immunological response that gives a slight advantage in fighting the virus. This may well have happened too, and the evidence suggests that a state of virus/host co-evolution has occurred, where all three have changed – the virus, rabbit behaviour and rabbit immunity. The change in immunity seems to have been least important of the three. This is illustrated by a difference in the situations in Europe and Australia. In Australia, highly attenuated, less lethal strains have replaced the more virulent original. In Europe, the two strains co-exist. This is because mosquitoes are less common in Europe, especially in Britain, and the disease is spread by fleas constantly throughout the year with less marked summer peaks. Myxomatosis is now permanently present at a low level in the wild rabbits of Europe, with occasional summer epidemics, particularly in France. During the epidemics, the mortality among the rabbits is much the same as it always was; the majority of rabbits have not developed significant immunity. This situation is almost precisely analogous to human smallpox prior to the widespread introduction of Jenner's vaccine.

The evidence relating to rabbits usefully illustrates what might happen to us. The most likely major infectious threat from a 'new' disease will come from a virus, as will be explained in more detail in Chapter Ten. Viruses have all the requirements for a novel source of epidemics: rapid mutation; ready transfer from animals; rapid transmission from person to person and via inanimate objects; as they may include an infectious period with no symptoms and often difficult to treat.

So what would happen if the equivalent of human myxomatosis were to develop; an illness with 99 per cent mortality and no known treatment? From the current world population of 6,478,889,071 (US Government Census figures), we would be left with a population of 64,800,000, give or take. Our own chances of survival do not look good. The first wave of such an outbreak would be catastrophic for the affected population. Would we really be reduced eventually to such fractions of our former numbers? Would we be powerless to prevent the second and subsequent waves of infection?

I would suggest not. What would initially protect us is the fact that we are far more heterogeneous, more different among ourselves, than rabbits. This applies to almost all aspects of the essence of being a rabbit and the essence of being a human. *Oryctolagus cuniculus* cannot successfully breed with wild rabbits or hares in countries where they exist. Remember that the Australian rabbit was derived from a population of only twenty-four. This means its genetic pool is limited; remember that these animals were introduced in most European countries and therefore with a similarly small genetic pool. Rabbits tend to interbreed within family units – sibling to sibling, parent to child – which, although it leads to a higher incidence of fatal mutations, means further limitations to the variability of the rabbit inheritance. Such behaviour in human populations is taboo. The chances, therefore, of a sub-group of humans happening to have relative immunity to any new agent are higher – although not absolute.

Even viruses to which there appears to be no useful immunity – HIV, for example – demonstrate considerable variability in their effects. Although it is believed that untreated infection is ultimately fatal in all victims, there are so-called Long Term Non-Progressors who seem to cohabit with the disease for prolonged periods. Furthermore, relative resistance to infection in some groups can occur. HIV needs to enter cells by a specific interaction like a lock and key between the virus and the white blood cell; some people appear to have a defective lock, or receptor, on their white blood cells which prevents the virus from entering and ultimately killing the cell. This mutation, which is called CCR5 delta 32, is not common, but it is remarkable that it existed before HIV ever became a widespread disease. There is absolutely no reason why such a mutation should not occur in the context of some other entirely new infection that we might face. Equally, there is absolutely no reason why it should.

Unlike rabbits, we do not rely on Darwinian selection, nor the chance of resistance to a new infection emerging in time for survival. However rapidly and catastrophically this imaginary epidemic might spread, there would inevitably be a lag period in which there would be opportunities for civil authorities throughout the world to institute public health measures. This might involve the closure of schools, theatres, cinemas and places of congregation, and the cordoning-off of infected areas. More extreme measures might include curfews; the shutting-down of airports and public transport; the introduction of martial law; and even the closure of hospitals, which sometimes serve as amplifiers of infection. There might also be fumigation and even destruction of affected premises. Most developed nations have plans for outbreaks with triggers for activating them; for example, twenty cases of a new illness would activate the Essex Health Protection Unit's Outbreak Control Plan. Of course, this supposes that our epidemic does not develop in Essex – around Stansted Airport, for instance – and that all the public health doctors, virologists, chief medical officers, GPs, nurses, policemen and so on, who would control the outbreak, are not already dead.

Herein lies a problem with control of a truly catastrophic outbreak, and one that would not require a mortality of 99 per cent to drop a fairly large spanner into the works. During the Great Plagues of history – where mortality stood at about 40 per cent – it is well documented that such social order as was available readily broke down in the worst years. There are eye-witness accounts of such chaos. Samuel Pepys, Daniel Defoe and Petrarch all give accounts of the shattered life of the Plague Years. In *The*

Decameron, Giovanni Boccaccio documented the consequences of the plague as it ravaged Florence in 1348. This is a fictional story of seven men and three women who escape the disease by fleeing to a villa outside the city. In his non-fictional introduction, Boccaccio gives a graphic description of the almost total disruption of any rule of law before this incurable disease, as well as the utter collapse of social conventions. As you will read, this shockingly included the most basic convention of all – the care of a mother for her children. Furthermore, you will read of an interesting behavioural modification concerning the morals of those women who survived. Rather like the rabbits, in fact. Is it possible that modern sexual morality is genetically determined by an epidemic of infectious disease which nearly killed our species?

The disorder was of a nature to defy . . . treatment, . . . almost all within three days from the appearance of the said symptoms, sooner or later, died . . .

  In which circumstances, not to speak of many others of a similar or even graver complexion, divers apprehensions and imaginations were engendered in the minds of such as were left alive, inclining almost all of them to the same harsh resolution, to wit, to shun and abhor all contact with the sick and all that belonged to them, thinking thereby to make each his own health secure. Among whom there were those who thought that to live temperately and avoid all excess would count for much as a preservative against seizures of this kind. Wherefore they banded together, and, dissociating themselves from all others, formed communities in houses where there were no sick, and lived a separate and secluded life, which they regulated with the utmost care, avoiding every kind of luxury, but eating and drinking very moderately of the most dèlicate viands and the finest wines, holding converse with none but one another, lest tidings of sickness or death should reach them, and diverting their minds with music and such other delights as they could devise. Others, the bias of whose minds was in the opposite direction, maintained, that to drink freely, frequent places of public resort, and take their pleasure with song and revel, sparing to satisfy no appetite, and to laugh and mock at no event, was the sovereign remedy for so great an evil: and that which they affirmed they also put in practice, so far as they were able, resorting day and night, now to this tavern, now to that, drinking with an entire disregard of rule or measure, and by preference making the houses of others, as it were, their inns, if they but saw in them aught that was particularly to their taste or liking; which they were readily able to do, because the owners, seeing death imminent, had become as reckless of their property as of their lives; so that most of the houses were open to all comers, and no distinction was observed between the stranger who presented himself and the rightful lord. Thus, adhering ever to their inhuman determination to shun the sick, as far as possible, they ordered their life. In this extremity of our city's suffering and tribulation the venerable authority of laws, human and divine, was abased and all but totally dissolved, for lack of those who should have administered and enforced them, most of whom, like the rest of the citizens, were either dead or sick, or so hard bested for servants that they were unable to execute any office; whereby every man was free to do what was right in his own eyes.

Some again, the most sound, perhaps, in judgment, as they were also the most harsh in temper, of all, affirmed that there was no medicine for the disease superior or equal in efficacy to flight; following which prescription a multitude of men and women, negligent of all but themselves, deserted their city, their houses, their estates, their kinsfolk, their goods, and went into voluntary exile, or migrated to the country parts, as if God in visiting men with this pestilence in requital of their iniquities would not pursue them with His wrath wherever they might be, but intended the destruction of such alone as remained within the circuit of the walls of the city; or deeming, perchance, that it was now time for all to flee from it, and that its last hour was come.

Tedious were it to recount, how citizen avoided citizen, how among neighbours was scarce found any that shewed fellow-feeling for another, how kinsfolk held aloof, and never met, or but

144

rarely; enough that this sore affliction entered so deep into the minds of men and women, that in the horror thereof brother was forsaken by brother, nephew by uncle, brother by sister, and oftentimes husband by wife; nay, what is more, and scarcely to be believed, fathers and mothers were found to abandon their own children, untended, unvisited, to their fate, as if they had been strangers. Wherefore the sick of both sexes, whose number could not be estimated, were left without resource but in the charity of friends (and few such there were), or the interest of servants, who were hardly to be had at high rates and on unseemly terms, and being, moreover, one and all, men and women of gross understanding, and for the most part unused to such offices, concerned themselves no further than to supply the immediate and expressed wants of the sick, and to watch them die; in which service they themselves not seldom perished with their gains. In consequence of which dearth of servants and dereliction of the sick by neighbours, kinsfolk and friends, it came to pass – a thing, perhaps, never before heard of – that no woman, however dainty, fair or well-born she might be, shrank, when stricken with the disease, from the ministrations of a man, no matter whether he were young or no, or scrupled to expose to him every part of her body, with no more shame than if he had been a woman, submitting of necessity to that which her malady required; wherefrom, perchance, there resulted in after time some loss of modesty in such as recovered. Besides which many succumbed, who with proper attendance, would, perhaps, have escaped death; so that, what with the virulence of the plague and the lack of due tendance of the sick, the multitude of the deaths, that daily and nightly took place in the city, was such that those who heard the tale – not to say witnessed the fact – were struck dumb with amazement. Whereby, practices contrary to the former habits of the citizens could hardly fail to grow up among the survivors.

Many passed from this life unregarded, and few indeed were they to whom were accorded the lamentations and bitter tears of sorrowing relations; nay, for the most part, their place was taken by the laugh, the jest, the festal gathering . . . The condition of the lower, and, perhaps, in great measure of the middle ranks, of the people shewed even worse and more deplorable; for, deluded by hope or constrained by poverty, they stayed in their quarters, in their houses, where they sickened by thousands a day, and, being without service or help of any kind, were, so to speak, irredeemably devoted to the death which overtook them. Many died daily or nightly in the public streets; of many others, who died at home, the departure was hardly observed by their neighbours, until the stench of their putrefying bodies carried the tidings; and what with their corpses and the corpses of others who died on every hand the whole place was a sepulchre.

It was the common practice of most of the neighbours, moved no less by fear of contamination by the putrefying bodies than by charity towards the deceased, to drag the corpses out of the houses with their own hands, aided, perhaps, by a porter, if a porter was to be had, and to lay them in front of the doors, where any one who made the round might have seen, especially in the morning, more of them than he could count; afterwards they would have biers brought up, or, in default, planks, whereon they laid them. Nor was it once or twice only that one and the same bier carried two or three corpses at once; but quite a considerable number of such cases occurred, one bier sufficing for husband and wife, two or three brothers, father and son, and so forth. And times without number it happened, that, as two priests, bearing the cross, were on their way to perform the last office for some one, three or four biers were brought up by the porters in rear of them, so that, whereas the priests supposed that they had but one corpse to bury, they discovered that there were six or eight, or sometimes more. Nor, for all their number, were their obsequies honoured by either tears or lights or crowds of mourners; rather, it was come to this, that a dead man was then of no more account than a dead goat would be to-day.

As consecrated ground there was not in extent sufficient to provide tombs for the vast multitude of corpses . . . , they dug, for each graveyard, as soon as it was full, a huge trench, in which they laid the corpses as they arrived by hundreds at a time, piling them up as merchandise is stowed in the hold of a ship, tier upon tier, each covered with a little earth, until the trench would hold no more.

It is not hard to imagine a situation where such mayhem might break out, even in the modern world. Imagine an epidemic which had even a 5 per cent mortality in London or New York. This would mean many thousands of deaths – if all of the population were affected equally, between 200,000 and 500,000. Suppose a vaccine were developed, or a treatment discovered, or, worse, a false rumour circulated that such measures were available to a privileged few. The institution where such stocks were believed to be held would be besieged; only martial law could control it. One only needs to observe the looting that occurred in New Orleans following the floods in 2005 to notice how thin is our veneer of civilisation. A cynical observer might also add that western civilisation is not, currently, at its most self-confident. Would a major epidemic be enough to topple it?

At the time of writing, the threat that concerns the world most is avian influenza. Pandemics of Influenza A have occurred throughout history at the rate of about three or four every century. We are well overdue. The mortality of those infected within the current outbreak is presently believed to be about 60 per cent. Superficially, it might seem that the risk of the violent disorder I am hypothesising would be assured with such figures. However, there are a number of caveats. First, so far avian influenza has yet, reliably and consistently, to be transmitted from human to human. There has been a possible case of transmission between people in Thailand in September 2004; however, this remains an isolated example. This explains the relatively low incidence. The numbers proven to have had the disease are presently relatively small, in the order of hundreds (although the probable number is higher; countries such as China have not been unduly forthcoming in providing figures). Those victims have principally been from South-East Asia, and have almost without exception had contact with fowl. There has been an outbreak in Holland, but once again the link with birds was clear cut as the only fatality was a vet who had visited a poultry farm; nor was it the same viral strain that is presently causing anxiety. There are particular scientific reasons for this, which I shall come to.

We could compare the current anxiety about bird flu to the 1918 pandemic. The speed with which the infection spread suggests that there was very little immunity to it, particularly in young adults, who were hardest hit. That virus had a particular predilection for lung tissue, which made younger people especially susceptible. The infection killed probably 40–50 million people worldwide; many more than the First World War. Would the same catastrophe overtake us this time, if the virus were to mutate in such a way that it spread among people?

We have already mentioned the affinity between the Horsemen of the Apocalypse: war, famine and pestilence canter almost in time, like some grotesque dressage event. In 1918, the world was recovering from the war to end all wars. Enormous social changes were taking place across the world; refugees were migrating to the United States and across Europe; millions of demobbed soldiers were returning home; the revolution was evolving in Russia. Epidemics thrive in such disrupted circumstances. It is believed by some experts that soldiers on the front line may have contracted avian flu from foraged poultry, and then it was carried home with them throughout the world.

That world – at least, in the West – is presently far more stable. Living conditions have improved for most. We live in less crowded houses; slums have been cleared; hygiene is better; we are healthier and more robust. You might assume that the mortality would be lower, although given the predilection of the 1918 strain for healthy young people, this remains an assumption. Conversely, the world is far more rapidly mobile today than in 1918. Flight in those days was a rarity and more or less a military venture; compare that to the present day, where at any given time over a million people may be airborne. Such promiscuity of travel might seem to guarantee rapid transmission of a highly infectious agent; particularly one that is at its most infectious before symptoms develop, and to which nobody has effective immunity.

Why did healthy young people preferentially die of influenza in 1917–18? Will the same thing happen with bird flu? We should pause a moment to consider the nature of immunity to influenza, because there is a peculiarity in relation to new disease strains that is contrary to received wisdom. Most of us think of immunity as an exclusively protective process. It is derived from the Greek for 'exemption from military service'. In the main, that assumption is correct. There are inherited defects of immunity that clearly demonstrate the functions of each branch and the perils of lacking them; suffice it to say that immunity to viruses requires antibodies and the production of potentially toxic chemicals called cytokines. Antibodies are proteins produced by white blood cells that are designed to precisely match and neutralise specific infections. If you have ever had flu, you will be familiar with the effects of cytokines. They actually cause your symptoms – the fever, headache and muscle pains of flu can be reproduced by injecting pure preparations of these fascinating and varied chemicals.

The main function of immunity is to select what is not you from what is you, and then destroy it. This is referred to as self and non-self. Production of antibodies and then cytokines is triggered by the detection of 'alien' non-self material within the body. There is a particular problem with viruses and self/non-self, because the virus incorporates itself into yourself. This poses an almost philosophical problem: if the virus is incorporated into your genes, what is you? Destruction of the virus may involve destruction of some of you. In some diseases, such as hepatitis B, the damage to the body is entirely self-directed. Friendly fire is the military euphemism.

The process is at its most efficient, with least collateral damage, where the antibody precisely recognises and matches the non-self material. Such a state will occur when the alien material has been met before, because white blood cells store the memory of the encounter indefinitely. A re-encounter will reawaken the stored memory. The brake to switch off the antibody/cytokine response is the elimination of the trigger. However, if the trigger and the antibody are poorly matched, the cascade of production of cytokines may be unstoppable. The result may be a massively

149

destructive process called a 'cytokine storm'. Any tissue may be destroyed – lungs, heart, brain, blood vessels. Because the primary route of infection for the 'Spanish' flu of 1918 was the lungs, most victims died of pneumonia. Because cytokine production wanes with age, the most vigorous 'cytokine storms' occurred in healthy young people. Basically, young people are better at killing themselves.

The strain of flu responsible for the 1918 outbreak has been recovered from victims in the Alaskan permafrost and identified by genetic sequencing. It is very different from the flu viruses that had been in circulation in the preceding decades. Understanding the principles of variation of the influenza virus is crucial to explaining the current anxiety about the disease, and the difficulties we face. To cause a fresh outbreak, the virus has to mutate. Enough immunity will develop in a community to control outbreaks if the virus does not change. Influenza can mutate in two distinct ways. The first is called genetic drift. This means that small changes occur – not enough to make the virus radically different, but enough to allow it to cause small, localised outbreaks. The other means of mutation is called genetic shift, and this is the more frightening of the two. Influenza is remarkable in that it has a 'segmented' genome. This means that it contains several – nine, in fact – parcels of genetic material that can be taken out and replaced like discs in a juke box. It is these discs that can be swapped when two infections occur within the same species. The term for this is 'genetic reassortment'. Say, for example, a pig already infected with pig flu encounters a duck with duck flu. The two viruses exchange discs. The next pig or duck in the chain will be infected with a totally new variant of flu, never before encountered, which is a hybrid of the two. The naming of the virus is exactly like selecting juke box discs: a letter and a number. Because we are particularly interested in the two parts of the virus that actually do the damage, naming refers to them. One is called the Haemagglutinin, the other Neuraminidase. These are abbreviated to their initials, and given an identification number, thus H5N1. More detailed naming would also include the year and site of identification.

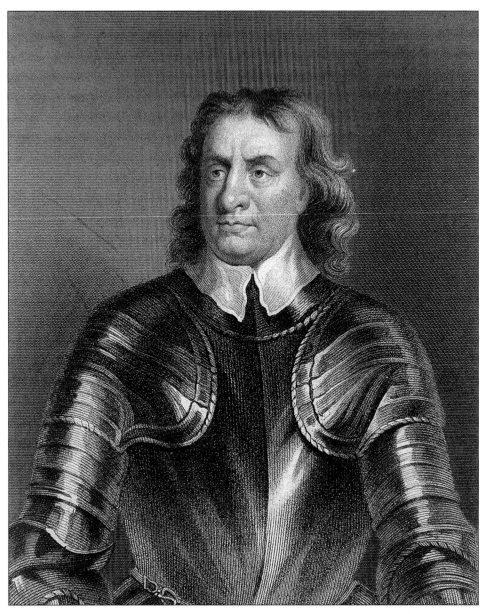

Oliver Cromwell, Lord Protector of England, was indirectly responsible for the worldwide spread of one of the most terrifying infectious diseases, Yellow Fever. Some might argue that his ultimate demise as a possible consequence of infection with another disease carried by mosquitoes – malaria – represented rough justice. The true cause of his death is debatable. *(The Wellcome Trust L0021169)*

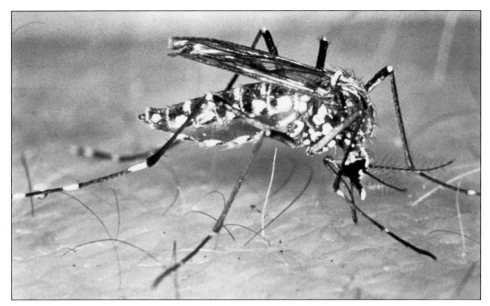

A female *Aedes aegyptii* mosquito, the vector of Yellow and Dengue Fevers. Only the females spread disease. The mosquito is the planet's most dangerous biting animal, with mortality from malaria exceeding that from shark bites by many orders of magnitude. Most of the world's emerging threats from infectious diseases are viral infections transmitted by biting insects. *(CDC/WHO)*

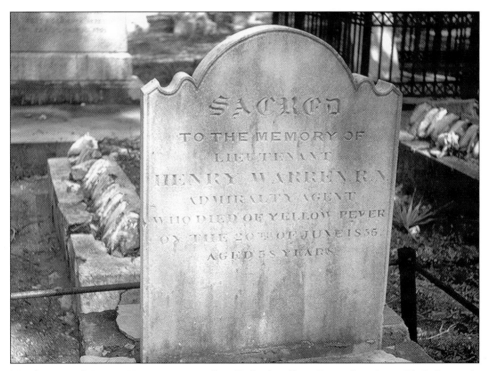

Tombstone of Henry Warren, RN, who died of Yellow Fever in 1855, Christiansted, St Croix, Virgin Islands. He might have blamed Oliver Cromwell for his demise. *(CDC)*

Henry VIII, an image which he carried in his own prayer book. He is plainly a sick man in this picture, with evidence of arthritis in his hands. The picture is also said to show evidence of syphilis in the distortion of the nose. Like Cromwell, the cause of his death is uncertain, but the belief that he died from syphilis is widely held. *(The Wellcome Trust L0010525)*

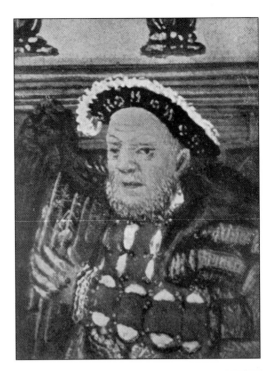

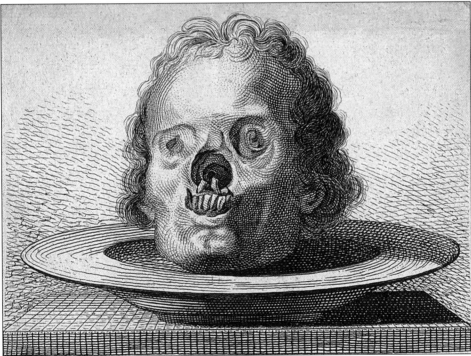

A line engraving of the preserved skull of a woman who had been suffering from syphilis and died in 1796. Syphilis was known as the Great Mimic, because of the huge variety of symptoms it could cause. We are witnessing a resurgence of this disease in the West, although fortunately it rarely progresses this far. *(The Wellcome Trust V0010536)*

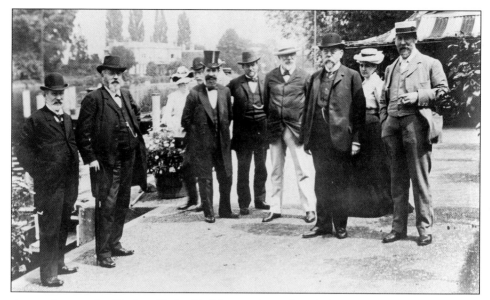

A rare photograph of Robert Koch (third from right) and Paul Ehrlich (extreme right) together, in Maidstone, Kent, UK in 1901 at the International Congress on Tuberculosis. It is impossible to overstate the influence that these two German scientists have had over the world of infectious diseases and immunology. *(The Wellcome Trust M0013275)*

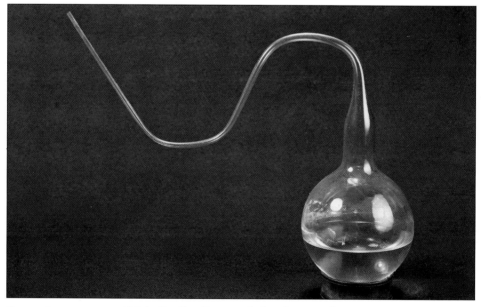

Pasteur's apparatus which finally disproved the theory of spontaneous generation. Troublesome insects such as lice and horseflies were held to arise under the correct atmospheric conditions from apparently inanimate matter, such as manure. The dogma had been under assault since the seventeenth century, but was not properly refuted until 1859. Oddly, the hypothesis has had something of a comeback related to the earliest origins of life; some chemicals are capable of spontaneous self-assembly in a manner which closely resembles RNA and DNA, the basic building blocks of life. *(The Wellcome Trust M0012521)*

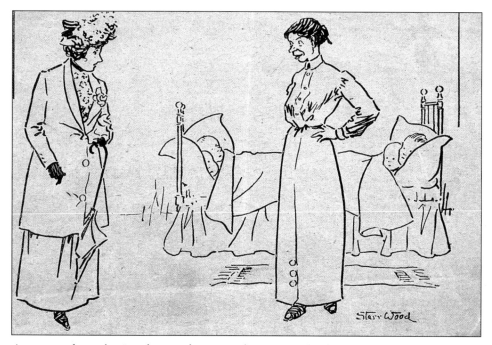

A cartoon from the *London Mail*, 23 October 1915. The futility of simple measures to prevent measles transmission was known even then, thirty-nine years before the virus was identified by Enders and Peebles, and twenty-five years before its route of spread was proven. Measles remains a highly infectious and lethal disease, and the world's leading cause of vaccine-preventable death, causing around 800,000 fatalities each year. There has been something of a resurgence of measles in some countries in the developed world as uptake of vaccination with MMR falls. Its prominent place among the Quiet Killers – number 6 in the league table of infectious killers – is forgotten at our peril. *(The Wellcome Trust V0015129)*

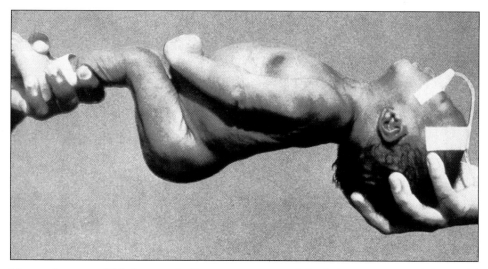

Neonatal tetanus. This is a tragically common cause of death in some parts of the world where immunisation is not universally provided. The organism responsible is *Clostridium tetani*. The infection usually enters via the stump of the umbilicus. *(CDC)*

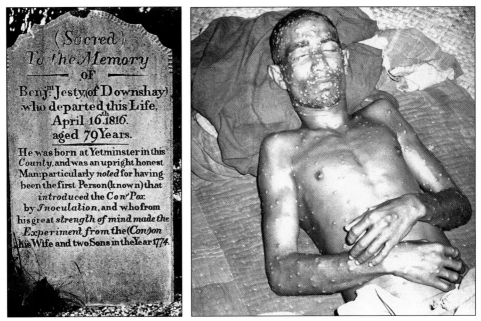

Above left: The grave of Benjamin Jesty, in Worth Matravers, Dorset. Jesty inoculated his family with cowpox to protect them from smallpox some years before Jenner introduced the practice. Jenner probably knew the story, and his genius lay in repeating the procedure in a meticulous and scientific manner. Scientists would probably not be allowed to perform such experiments today. *(The Wellcome Trust V0018800)*

Above right: Smallpox in an adult from Bangladesh. This is, surprisingly, not the most severe variant of the disease. The rash usually arises around the mouth and throat, at which point the disease is at its most infectious. Characteristically, blisters spread from the face to the trunk, arms and legs in an order which distinguishes the disease from chickenpox. Mortality was traditionally in the order of 30 per cent; whether this would remain true in a modern outbreak in an unvaccinated population with no natural immunity from circulating natural disease is debatable. *(CDC/WHO; Stanley O. Foster MD, MPH)*

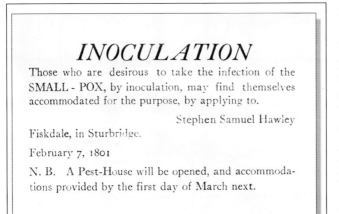

Smallpox inoculation sign, 1801. Edward Jenner is widely accredited with pioneering the vaccine that ultimately eradicated smallpox from the world. Whether this is accurate or not is open to debate; Jenner was not the first to vaccinate with cowpox. By the date of this poster, 100,000 people had been vaccinated in England. *(CDC)*

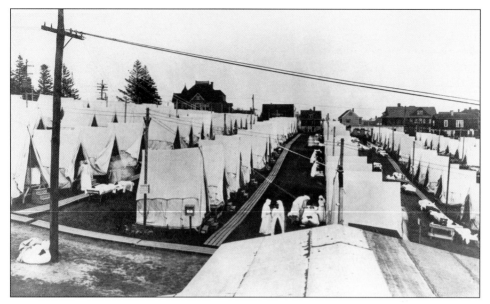

Influenza tents from Lawrence, Massachusetts, 1918. Such encampments were set up to nurse and isolate victims of the Great Influenza Pandemic of 1918. The death toll was enormous, amounting to 20–50 million with 675,000 in the United States alone. Many fear that the world may face such a threat again. *(CDC)*

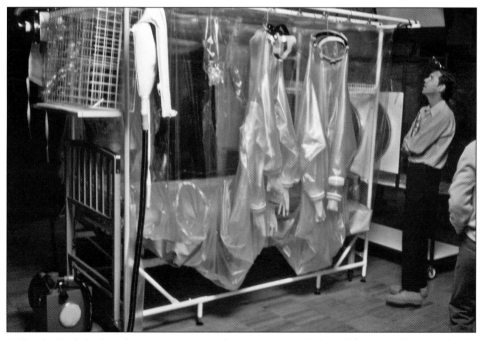

A Trexler bed. Such isolation tents are used to protect medical staff from viral haemorrhagic fevers, such as Lassa, Ebola and Marburg. These viruses are present in body fluids of infected victims; as the means of death is usually bleeding, there is a very real risk of nurses and doctors acquiring the illness. The patient may expect a prolonged stay in such a bed before recovery, unless death intervenes. *(CDC/Dr Lyle Conrad)*

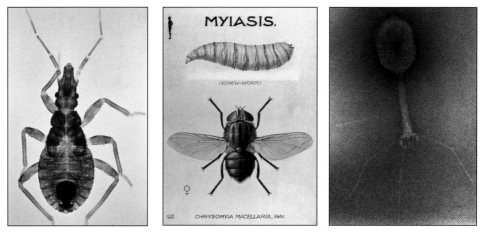

Above left: The reduviid or kissing bug. Also known as the assassin bug, this charming insect transmits the agent of Chagas' Disease by defecating into the site of its own bite. The parasite thus inoculated, *Trypanosoma cruzi*, is toxic to nerve cells in the intestine and heart; death is by heart failure or aspiration of stomach contents into the lungs. *(CDC/Donated by the WHO)*

Above centre: Screw-worm larvae. These ultimately hatch into the strangely beautiful metallic flies. Like the maggots they resemble, they eat meat. Unlike maggots, they also eat living flesh and may kill by burrowing through the nose and into the brain. *(The Wellcome Trust V0022565)*

Above right: Transmission electron micrograph of bacteriophage. These remarkable and fascinating viruses may offer some hope in combating the scourge of resistant bacteria. *(The Wellcome Trust B0004775)*

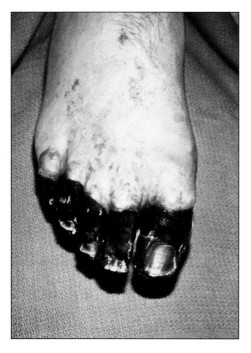

Plague foot. The gangrene of the toes explains why infection with *Yersinia pestis* was known as the Black Death. Cases still occur worldwide, although nowadays it is treatable with simple antibiotics. *(CDC/William Archibald)*

Our new hybrid pig–duck virus may not matter to humans. Apart from the economic consequences of a flu outbreak in what may be farmed animals, the virus may be restricted to the original animal species that it infected. The reason for this is that the virus can only bind to specific conformations of cell. The cells have markers on them, which act as locks for the viral key. These are called sialic acid residues. It is the 'H' or Haemagglutinin component which binds to the residue. Different species have different residues; thus, duck virus cannot usually infect horses. Furthermore, within species there may be different residues in each tissue. The 1918 outbreak was so successful because it bound to residues in human lung tissue, which made it readily transmissible by inhalation. At present, H5N1 binds to the wrong residues, which is why human–human transmission is not happening consistently. Close physical contact of the type that might result from butchering poultry seems to be needed to catch the disease. This is how the original outbreak began in Hong Kong in 1997. There were four proven human cases; three died. All had contact with chickens.

Here's where the danger is. Supposing a pig has a variant of flu which has the right key for binding to human lung sialic acid residues. This is reasonable, because pigs are more closely related to humans than chickens; the sialic acid residues in their lungs are more like ours. This particular virus causes minor or trivial or no illness in humans. The pig becomes infected with flu from another species, which has the capacity to cause severe illness but does not bind to the right sialic acid residues in human lungs. The two viruses do their juke box swap. Now we have a virus which has all the components to do real harm to humans. It has the right Haemagglutinin for binding to human sialic acid residues and the right Neuraminidase to do the damage. The virus can infect pig, or duck, or human. As far as our immunity is concerned, this is a completely new virus. Human myxomatosis. Outbreak. Pandemic.

The present – and future – situation is slightly more dangerous than this might imply. The difference between the virus that can and cannot bind to human sialic acid residues may be very small indeed. Only a very simple mutation, of the sort caused by genetic drift, might be enough to transform bird flu into human flu. When we reproduce our cells for growth, our cells have extremely accurate mechanisms for ensuring that their copies are faithful and accurate. Viruses are far sloppier: errors creep in all the time. Given the reproduction rate of the virus, the prevalence in the bird population and the number of birds in the world, it is statistically only a matter of time before this mutation arises. Some scientists are convinced that a bird flu pandemic among humans is therefore inevitable. There have already been some alarming signs that we are well along this road. Initially, H5N1 was carried by wild migratory birds, and shed in their droppings. It did not actually make them ill. In 2003, that changed – wildfowl began to die. For this to happen, the virus must have mutated. Does this mean the pandemic is inevitable? By the time you read this, we may know the answer.

A really worrying development would be the transmission of H5N1 between mammals of the same species – cats, say. In 2004, tigers in Bangkok Zoo were fed with H5N1-infected, slaughtered chickens. Over forty big cats died. That is tragic enough, but the really scary part of this outbreak is that some of the tigers had not eaten the chicken. If tigers can pass the virus between one another, why not humans? The transmission between cats has been reproduced experimentally among domestic cats in the laboratory, in the Erasmus Medical Centre in Rotterdam. A dead cat infected with H5N1 has recently been found in Germany. Given that there has been a hint of transmission between family members in Thailand already, we have every reason to be anxious.

Are we all going to die? The good news for us is that nobody really knows, least of all the experts. At a lecture at London's prestigious Royal College of Physicians a few years ago, at the height of the scare over mad cow disease, the government's leading expert in the field gave a talk, most impressive in its presentation, argument and scientific detail, which predicted anywhere between 10,000 and 1 million victims in Britain. It was claimed that hospices for the terminally ill would be required in every town and village.

There are similar predictions about the likely mortality from a pandemic, and how it may be controlled. Once again, we are not rabbits, passively awaiting our fate. There is a treatment for avian flu, which interferes with the destructive processes of the infection. It blocks the action of the N part of H5N1, the Neuraminidase. It is this enzyme which is responsible for the virus particle exploding out of the cell and allowing it to spread to other tissues. In fact, there are two of these drugs which block Neuraminidase. One is called oseltamivir and the other zanamivir. The latter is less useful because it has to be inhaled. The pharmaceutical company which makes the former is working flat out to meet demand and has asked for help. The really good news is that resistance has already emerged, in outbreaks among children in Thailand and Japan. In the first wave of any pandemic, such drugs will be absolutely crucial in reducing mortality. Unlike rabbits, we can also vaccinate ourselves. There are problems with vaccines for the bird flu outbreak. Nobody knows for certain which exact strain is going to cause the epidemic, and stockpiling a virus in advance may prove pointless if it turns out to be the wrong one. The virus which caused the outbreak in Holland in 2003 was not H5N1, but H7N7. It killed a vet and resulted in the deaths of millions of chickens. Suppose we switch the world's total vaccine-generating capacity to H5N1, only for an alternative strain to emerge? What if the virus has mutated so much by the time it causes a pandemic that the vaccine is useless? Some scientists believe that a poorly matched vaccine is actually worse than no vaccine at all, because it may suppress the symptoms yet cause people – and birds, if they are vaccinated – to become carriers, increasing the spread of the virus.

There may also be a problem with generating the right vaccine in any event. The reason we know so much about influenza is that it was one of the first viruses to be grown successfully in embryonated hens' eggs. The virus is still manufactured in those eggs. You can see a problem here. Hens are birds. This is a bird virus. Our vaccine may kill the embryos, and vaccine production may fail. We may have to resort to genetic engineering to produce the right vaccine.

How would this work? The genetic material of influenza virus is RNA, the precursor of DNA. It is a fiddly business, but it is possible to work out the code of the RNA and find out which bit does the damage to the hens' eggs. You can then design a tool which splices out the toxic part, and then grow that in eggs. As an added twist, you can also splice in a bit of virus that reproduces very efficiently to improve your yield. This is called reverse genetic engineering. As you can imagine, it doesn't happen overnight – there would be a lag between deciding which virus you needed to vaccinate against, and producing enough vaccine to be useful.

What would be the ultimate mortality of an avian flu pandemic? Modelling based on the best available data now puts it at about 1 per cent of the world's population, in a period lasting about six months. There are huge numbers of mights and maybes and ifs in these sorts of projections. You do not need to be a genius mathematician to calculate the final toll with a global population of 6.5 billion. The numbers will probably not be evenly distributed. It is almost impossible to think of a means of transmission of an infection that will result in exposure of 100 per cent of humans. Isolated, low-density rural populations will inevitably be less likely to be affected than urban ones. Unprepared societies may be more severely struck than those with stockpiles of antivirals and vaccines; sadly, this probably means the usual suspects in the developing world.

It is worth noting here, however, that some of the great epidemics of history vanished without conscious or effective public health management, or vaccines, or antibiotics. TB was beginning to disappear long before the introduction of BCG or successful drug treatments, a trend we now fear may be reversing. The plague has died out in Europe. Why it should have done so is something of a mystery, and it is therefore worth discussion within the context of diseases that might kill us all, on the grounds that it is already the disease that has come closest. Disappearance of the Black Death was not due to attenuation of the bacillus. Plague is caused by a bacterium, described in detail below. Bacteria are less susceptible to spontaneous attenuation than viruses, on account of their generally lower rate of mutation, and in the case of plague the fact that it can 'escape' to its animal reservoir. In Africa, Asia and South America the disease remains endemic and is just as lethal to the unvaccinated as it was in 1348 and 1665. It occasionally still causes epidemics. Infection control practices including gowns, masks and isolation remain just as important as they ever were. In the modern era, there are vaccines, there are rat control programmes and there are effective antibiotics, but the plague bacillus has not changed its spots.

As we have said, plague is caused by a bacterium, *Yersinia pestis*, discovered simultaneously in 1894 in Switzerland and Japan by Alexander Yersin and Shibasaburo Kitasato respectively. It grows readily in the laboratory without special growth requirements, although it prefers lower temperatures than many bacteria, growing optimally at about 28°C. Colonies of the bacterium are said to have a beaten-copper appearance on agar plates. Plague has two principal routes of transmission to humans, and causes at least two distinct pictures of disease. The bacterium hitches a ride in the intestines of the rat flea. Only a certain kind of flea called *Oropsylla* will do, and the flea is broadly restricted to certain mammals. In the wild, the plague may be harboured by rabbits, hares, marmots, prairie dogs and squirrels. Occasional transmission to humans – fur trappers, for instance – may occur from these animals. This is the so-called 'campestral' or 'sylvatic' route. The flea may also transmit to other rodent species with closer contact to urban humans. These include guinea pigs, hamsters and the black rat *Rattus rattus*. Domestic cats and dogs may also serve as a residence for the flea, or the prey rodent may transmit its fleas to the predator. In sufficiently heavy infestations of fleas, where humans have close enough contact with these species for long enough, the bacterium can transmit to the blood-stream of victims. Bubonic plague will result. The buboes are swollen, ulcerating and dead, necrotic lymph glands. Death is from overwhelming blood infection – septicaemia – as the rapidly reproducing bacillus spills over from these dying tissues. The fingers, toes and even the nose may also die before the victim, turning these peripheral organs black – hence, the Black Death.

By contrast, pneumonic plague may be spread from lung to lung. It is coughed up and inhaled by the next victim. It requires no flea or rat intermediary, although it can be transmitted to humans from animals with pneumonic plague – domestic cats, for example. Pneumonic plague may derive from bubonic, septicaemic plague. Once the illness becomes septicaemic, it is no respecter of tissues; the lungs are as likely to be affected as any other tissue. This is known as secondary pneumonic plague. Primary pneumonic plague, by contrast, arises from direct inhalation. The brain and throat (pharynx) may also be affected in secondary disease; the first being significant as it will cause rapidly fatal meningitis, the second because pharyngeal plague is highly infectious.

Most of the European plagues were principally rat-borne and bubonic in form, with a smaller proportion of secondary pneumonic cases. However, at least three of the major plagues of history changed from bubonic – that is, rat–flea–human transmission – to pneumonic – human–human transmission. These were the Plague of Justinian in AD 540–90, the Black Death of 1348–50 and the Great Plague of the mid-seventeenth century. The hallmark of this metamorphosis is a sudden increase in the number of victims. In the Plague of London between July 1665 and the third week of September, the weekly Bills of Mortality increased from 100 to 7,000 per week. Such a massive surge in the rate of transmission cannot be explained by a sudden increase in the number of rats or fleas. Some authorities believe this represented a change in the virulence of *Yersinia pestis*. This may be possible, and will be discussed in more detail below. However, you do not need to invoke sophisticated alterations in the nature of the infection to explain transition from rat–flea–human transmission to explosive pneumonic. It is entirely possible that the pandemic emerged more as a matter of mathematics than of genetic alteration to the bacillus. Epidemics may behave rather like a nuclear bomb. Once a critical mass of fissile material is reached, instability and explosion result. The critical mass in the case of the plague is the proportion of victims with the more infectious pneumonic variety of the disease. Initially, these would probably have been secondary cases, but as the pandemic evolved, an increasing number would have contracted primary pneumonic plague that readily transmitted to the next victim.

Whether or not the explosive transmission of pneumonic plague was a purely mathematical phenomenon, it is entirely possible – likely, even – that *Yersinia* changed itself during this transition. This may have been a consequence of the fascinating phenomenon of 'Quorum Sensing', mentioned in the introduction. I have said that bacteria are less susceptible to mutation than viruses. In fact, this is not entirely true. Bacteria can spontaneously mutate. They are exceptionally effective at transferring genetic information between one another, splicing and swapping whole genes. The difference between viruses and bacteria in this respect is one of evolutionary pressure. As a general rule, an encounter with a virus leads to permanent immunity. Unless severe and debilitating illness like cancer or AIDS intervenes, each morbid encounter (should you survive) with a particular viral species, whether it be smallpox, chickenpox or SARS, will be your last. This is not so with most bacterial infections. One staphylococcal boil provides comparatively little protection from the next. There is thus little incentive for the bacterium to mutate. This state of affairs changes when, for example, antibiotics are entered into the equation. Bacteria with resistance mutations are then at a reproductive advantage; mutation is encouraged. Viruses need no such encouragement. They have to mutate to survive.

Bacteria also can – and do – become more or less dangerous, changing their virulence. *Streptococcus pyogenes* is an unpleasant bacterium which can cause severe and even fatal infections of flesh. It is also capable of causing longer-term complications after infection. Scarlet fever, destruction of heart valves, kidney damage, arthritis and brain damage can all follow streptococcal infection. For some poorly understood reason, *Streptococcus pyogenes* is a far less unpleasant infection than it used to be. Rheumatic fever is a complication of infection with that bacterium. At one time, it was one of the commonest causes of damaged heart valves in the western world; now, it is rarely encountered. This leopard has changed its spots. While we know that *Yersinia pestis* is behaving much as it ever did in endemic areas of the world, it may have altered its virulence in Europe in the seventeenth century, when it finally vanished.

There are other means by which bacteria can change their virulence. Some modify their behaviour according to the tissues in which they find themselves. *Listeria monocytogenes* is an excellent example; it does not produce its toxins until it has safely penetrated the interior of a cell. Other *Yersinia* species do the same. It is entirely plausible that a combination of these factors was responsible for the rise and fall of the pneumonic plague. *Yersinia pestis* (perhaps through Quorum Sensing) switches on different toxins when it invades lung tissues in secondary pneumonic plague. These toxins permit lung to lung transmission more readily, with the consequence that there is an explosion of primary pneumonic plague. This eruption subsides only when the whole susceptible population has died, or when the bacterium downregulates its virulence.

So why did both pneumonic and bubonic plague die out? Pneumonic plague probably behaved rather like myxomatosis among rabbits; it simply killed every infected and susceptible person. Rates of mortality in the order of 90 per cent were certainly recorded. The initial outbreak of plague in the Chinese province of Hubei in 1334 claimed up to 90 per cent of the population, an estimated 5 million people. Remember the words of the plague nursery rhyme, 'Ring-a-Ring o' Roses' – 'A-tishoo, a-tishoo, / We all fall down'. Place the emphasis on the second word of the last line, 'all', and the meaning changes in a most sinister way. Once the threshold of pneumonic plague sufferers fell below the critical level again, the epidemic switched back to the less infectious bubonic form. This also died out. Why this should have happened is the subject of some debate. We shall probably never know. Mass infections are like empires. The causes of their decline are often hard to pinpoint.

Some believe that the black rat disappeared, taking its infected fleas with it. Rather like the replacement of the red squirrel by the grey in Europe, its habitat was taken over by the brown rat *Rattus norvegicus*, which is a host to different non-plague-bearing fleas. The problem with this hypothesis is that the data do not fully support it. First, the brown rat does not compete for territory with the black. Second, nor has the black rat entirely disappeared from countries from where the plague has. Third, in the Black Death of 1348–50, the population of Iceland was reduced by a half to one third. There were said to be no rats in Iceland at that time; they were not introduced until the nineteenth century. Finally, the plague bacillus is as lethal to the rat as it is to the human. Not every plague was associated with finding an excess of dead rats.

We should recall, with some trepidation, that the period between the Black Death of 1348 and the Great Plague of 1665 is 317 years. No sophisticated public health measure or vaccine caused its disappearance. If this is the 'periodicity' of the epidemic, then we are due for another. Of course, this time we would have vaccines, rat control, public health alerts and effective antibiotics – common preparations such as tetracycline are effective – but there is no guarantee that the form a new plague would take would be the same as the last time. We don't know for certain why the Great Plagues started, killed so many, then disappeared. We aren't even certain that they were caused by *Yersinia pestis*.

The evidence is conflicting. A team from France claimed to have detected DNA from the plague bacillus in the dental pulp of a medieval victim in Montpellier. Other teams have not been able to repeat this finding. Some scientists have observed the behaviour of rats and fleas in areas where plague remains endemic, like India. They claim that the circumstances favouring transmission could never have occurred in northern Europe. Various alternative suggestions have been made for other agents that may have caused the plagues. A virus very like the one which causes Ebola fever (see Chapter Eight) has been mooted by some. The relatively long incubation period of the Black Death (up to thirty days) and its rapid spread support this theory to some extent. Tantalisingly, genes which confer partial immunity to Ebola are more common in Europeans than other races. Anthrax is another hypothesis; *Bacillus anthracis* has certainly been found in some plague pits. Hanta virus – a very unpleasant lung infection inhaled in dried rodent droppings, which caused an outbreak in the United States in 1993 – has been another candidate. The problem is that the final consequences of severe and overwhelming infection – collapse, pneumonia, necrosis of the extremities, uncontrollable bleeding – are shared by many illnesses. My own feeling is that we need look no further than *Y. pestis*. The presence of buboes in the early phases of the disease, followed by the explosive spread of the more infectious pulmonary form, fits the data better than any other.

Our Quiet Killers comprise viruses, bacteria, fungi, protozoa, parasites and prions. Unlike all the others, with the exception of the mysterious prions, viruses are incomplete. They cannot reproduce without invading a cell. As they do so, they convert the machinery of the tissues they invade into highly efficient cloning machines. A single virus in a cell can produce many thousands of progeny to be released and infect a new host or new cells in the same victim. The other Quiet Killers, although they are capable of phenomenal rates of reproduction, are relatively hampered by the fact that they have to produce their own factories to reproduce themselves. This gives viruses enormous advantages in terms of rapid, epidemic transmission. They are also tiny and therefore easily spread by droplets and casual contact. The largest viruses infecting humans are the pox viruses, which are just about on the verge of being visible under a light microscope. Bacteria are many thousands of times bigger; fungi larger yet; parasites and protozoa vast by microbial standards.

As we have already said, most importantly viruses have enormous capacity for mutation. This is more particularly true of viruses like influenza, which are composed of the slightly more unstable RNA. Your cells will not tolerate errors in reproduction. All of the other Quiet Killers, with the exception of prions, have DNA as their basic genetic code. DNA is more stable and less error-prone during replication. Bacteria use DNA as their genetic material. They are not therefore capable of the rates of mutation or of transmission to present a serious enough challenge to the majority of humans. The plague – caused by a bacterium – was able to kill so many because nobody knew how it was transmitted and there were no vaccines or effective treatments; the same would not apply today.

Supposing my assumption that we will probably never encounter a totally new infection proves incorrect, is there anything else that can be done about it, apart from quarantine, martial law and mass panic? As I have said, the most likely new threat will be a virus. There is, in fact, a drug which could save some of us. Cidofovir is an agent principally used for unusual viral infections in AIDS and in patients with cancers. It seems to be active against a variety of viruses; we have every reason to suppose it might be active against a number of new viral agents. Ribavirin is another antiviral drug that has activity against multiple viral species; we may reasonably hope that this will also be of benefit.

So, is there an infectious disease that could kill us all? It depends what you mean by 'us all'. There are agents that could do so – you could hold in a small glass test tube enough toxin from the bacterium *Clostridium botulinum* to kill every man, woman and child on the planet. The mechanism by which the toxin acts is universal; it would be almost impossible for any of us to have immunity to the poison. The difficulty with botulinum toxin is delivering it to enough people. But a Quiet Killer that could wipe us all out? I do not believe that an infection could emerge that could exterminate every last human on the planet. There is, though, probably a threshold somewhere between order and chaos in the developed world, where sufficiently prevalent disease could lead to the fall of our civilisation, much as it did to the Romans. *Sic*(k) *transit gloria mundi.*

EIGHT

Repellent and Morbid
Horrible Rarities

Some diseases are repulsive by their appearance or the way in which they make you ill. They have the power to shock and repel out of proportion to their rarity. This chapter examines a few, such as the nose-burrowing larva of *Cochliomya hominivorax*; the disfiguring espundia variant of Leishmaniasis; and the viral haemorrhagic fevers which cause fatal internal bleeding.

There was an argument that was used by Victorian philosophers to attempt to prove that the universe is structured and organised according to a divine plan. Imagine walking through a deserted field. In doing so, you notice an object on the ground. You pick it up, and discover it to be a watch. From the fact of its being a complex item with an obvious function, you deduce that it must have had a purposeful creator. Imagine and compare the structure of the eye. It is, of course, many orders of magnitude more sophisticated than a watch. Therefore, the existence of a creator of the universe is confirmed; and that confirmation is supported by a force of argument with at least the same order of magnitude. Observing some of the nastier members of the Quiet Killers, you might be forgiven for pursuing a similar argument to this watchmaker hypothesis. Some of these diseases are so unpleasant that they seem to imply a malevolent creator – the horrible watchmaker. This analogy is of course a slightly facetious one; evolution is not concerned with benevolence or malignity, but is 'blind'. And the watchmaker argument has been effectively demolished by various evolutionary biologists, such as Richard Dawkins. But why are there such vindictively horrible diseases? What has humankind done to deserve them?

Most diseases, infectious or otherwise, can cause unpleasant symptoms. That's why they are called diseases. A heart attack may be associated with severe pain and a terrifying sense of impending mortality. The pain of a kidney stone is said to be almost unbearable. Many cancers have appalling symptoms associated with them. Nonetheless, in my experience there is something about the more lurid types of infections that causes visceral revulsion in some observers. Perhaps it is the involvement of an external agent. Becoming 'ill' is one thing; being attacked by some nasty bug is another, particularly if it is big enough to be visible to the naked eye.

The apparent difference of the involvement of an external agent between the diseases listed above and the Quiet Killers is an arbitrary one; heart disease, kidney stones and even some cancers all have an infectious component. However, these illnesses lack the apparently single-minded malignity of some of the more exotic and unusual illnesses that prey on man. Take, for instance, the screw-worms. These are the larvae of the strangely beautiful so-called metallic flies, the Calliphoridae. They are known as metallic because of their livid, iridescent blue and green body parts. Their beauty is misleading; in their behaviour, they could have sprung straight from the movie *Alien*. The flies readily justify their inclusion among the Quiet Killers, as invasion by these peculiar insects can be lethal to humans.

Screw-worms are divided into two types: Old World and New World. The technical, biological names of the flies as adults are *Chrysomya bezziana* and *Cochliomyia hominivorax* respectively. The latter name may provide a hint about the nature of the beast – *hominivorax* is Latin for 'man-eater'. New World screw-worms are now confined to Mexico, Guatemala and Belize. They once occurred in the southern and central United States, but were eradicated there by a control programme which involved swamping their breeding territory with infertile males; an outbreak in Libya in 1991 was contained by the same method. Old World metallic flies occur in tropical Africa, the Indian sub-continent, and most of South-East Asia including China, the Philippines and Papua New Guinea. There are tiny differences in appearance between Old World and New

World metallic flies and their larvae, but otherwise they behave and appear more or less the same. It is their larvae, the juvenile worm-like forms, that concern us as predators of man. Screw-worms are like maggots, and they feed on flesh. Unlike most maggots, these larvae have a particular and specific dietary quirk. The flesh they feed on has to be living.

Female metallic flies like to lay their eggs in old wounds, scabs and sores. They will also use healthy skin, especially the moister areas around the mouth, nose, eyes and vagina. They sometimes also use the umbilicus of new-born babies as a hatchery. Batches of up to 500 eggs are laid. These hatch within 24 hours, and proceed to form a voracious gang which burrows ever deeper into the living tissue. Considerable tissue destruction may result; the damaged areas are thus highly prone to infection with bacteria and fatal sepsis may result. The resulting ulcers may be foul-smelling and putrescent. After about four to eight days, the larvae, now engorged with flesh, reach maturity and emerge from the passages they have dug, drop to the ground, bury themselves and form pupae. In warm conditions, a fertile fly may emerge after seven to ten days, but in cooler weather they may hide in the earth for weeks. Just to emphasise its charming nature, adult metallic flies also feed on excreta, decomposing corpses and rotting matter. This is not just a matter of aesthetics; a larva burrowing through tissue that has been contaminated by the faecally contaminated feet of its mother is far more likely to leave deadly suppuration in its tracks.

These screw-worm infections can cause excruciating pain, misery, permanent disfigurement and death. The larvae may be very numerous. One patient with an Old-World worm infection of the nose had 385 larvae removed over a nine-day period. Screw-worms may even burrow through the bone of the skull, destroying the palate, impairing speech and causing fatal meningitis. The larvae can – and should – be killed with chloroform or ethanol applied to the affected areas; however, in advanced cases complex and radical surgery may be necessary. Screw-worm infections also have major economic consequences in rural economies, because they affect livestock like goats, sheep and horses in just the same way as humans.

Rather like screw-worm, the potentially horrific disease Leishmaniasis has New World and Old World variants. There are a number of manifestations of the disease, from simple, diminutive ulcers the size of a small coin to a frequently fatal condition called visceral leishmaniasis or Kala-azar (which means 'black sickness'). In between these two extremes is a grotesque and disfiguring condition of the face called espundia. *Leishmania* is a parasite transmitted to humans by the bites of tiny sandflies. The milder version of the disease is well known to soldiers who have served in desert areas; Montgomery's Eighth Army would have known it as Biskra button, Delhi boil or Aleppo evil. Ironically for the so-called Desert Rats, rodents are a reservoir of the disease. Leishmaniasis was named after the British surgeon Sir William Leishman (1865–1926) who first identified the parasite; however, the disease has been known since ancient times, and indeed a form of immunisation was traditionally carried out against the disease by nomadic desert peoples who would allow their children to contract mild leishmaniasis by exposing them to sandflies. These small, short-lived insects are the vector and they transmit the disease between animals, including us.

Espundia is a variant of skin infection with one of the sub-species of New World *Leishmania*, usually *braziliensis*. The horribly mutilating disease may develop a few days after the initial infection, or, cruelly, up to twenty-five years later. *Leishmania* parasites spring up at some distance from the initial bite site. Ulcers begin to appear on the nose and mouth. Usually, they are on the edges of the lips or the nostril, but sometimes they can be in the mouth, the windpipe, the eyes or the genitals. The tip of the nose may disintegrate, leading to a characteristic appearance of 'tapir nose'. The nose may completely block off. The whole of the face around the mouth and nose may become horribly scarred; further bacterial infections may develop and sometimes breathing and swallowing may be so disrupted that food is aspirated into the lungs with a consequent fatal pneumonia.

For sheer repulsiveness, it is hard to beat South American Trypanosomiasis, also known as Chagas' Disease. By the standards of the Quiet Killers, this is an advanced and sophisticated organism. It is a parasite which enters the body through the bloodstream, aided by a peculiar and unpleasant yet strangely beautiful insect. It causes disease in humans by settling in nerve and heart cells. Infection of the heart causes this organ to fail; in countries like Brazil, it has become one of the leading reasons for people to need heart transplantation. *Trypanosoma cruzi*, the parasite involved, has a particular predilection for the muscle cells. It frequently invades the muscles of the gullet, or oesophagus. This organ, when infected, ceases to function properly. The coordination of swallowing is lost and death may occur from stomach contents being regurgitated and inhaled into the lungs. Infection of the colon may lead to severe and prolonged constipation, and the colon may occasionally twist and rupture. This grotesque means of death finds a strange and scatological parallel in the route which *T. cruzi* uses to enter the body. The parasite enters by means of the bite of a deadly insect, known, appropriately enough, as the Assassin Bug. This large animal, which is about 4cm long, is also known as the Reduviid, triatomine or kissing bug. There are various species, going by the Latin names *Panstrongylus megistus*, *Triatoma infestans*, *Triatoma braziliensis* and *Triatoma pseudomaculata*. This bug lurks in the rafters and cracks of traditionally made huts in rural and semi-rural areas of South America. It emerges at night to take a blood meal from the sleeping inhabitants of the hut. Unlike the mosquito, it does not simply release its infected load through its mouthparts; that would be far too straightforward. Instead, in a strange and vindictive dance, it reverses its posture over the site of its bite and defecates into the wound. Along with its stool, the parasite is able to slip into the bloodstream. Although this is not the sole route by which it can infect – there have been outbreaks related to sugar cane juice – this is by far the most common. Suspected victims may have to suffer one final indignity prior to treatment, a test known as xenodiagnosis. This means that they have to be bitten by the Assassin Bug once more. Uninfected laboratory insects are used; thirty days later they are dissected and the presence of trypanosomes in their intestines proves the diagnosis.

Loa loa is a parasite of man that occurs in West and Central Africa. It is transmitted by the day-biting fly *Chrysops*. The fact of its biting by day is of interest to more than entomologists; the parasite is at its most active in the bloodstream at midday, to synchronise with the bite of the fly. This synchrony allows it to spread to its next victim. Adult loa loa, whose females may be up to 70mm long, wander round the tissues just underneath the skin, like the lost souls of the damned. These worms may live for seventeen years or more. The commonest symptoms are the so-called Calabar swellings. These are transient, itchy lumps which may appear on any part of the body, but usually present on the ankles and wrists. They probably represent an allergic reaction to a worm passing through; they last a few hours or sometimes days. Sometimes worms may actually be seen passing under the skin. They move quickly and their tracks may be visible only for 15–20 minutes. This may happen around the eye, as may Calabar swellings. However, most repugnantly, the worm itself may actually migrate through the clear jelly inside the eyeball. Death may occur in loa loa; usually from intense scarring of the heart muscles, or sometimes from an infection of the brain, which may paradoxically and cruelly develop after treatment.

*   *   *

The viral haemorrhagic fevers (VHF) are a group of illnesses that cause no small consternation among doctors concerned with infectious diseases. They are rare yet cause outbreaks, usually in Africa, with a high mortality. There are a number of them; Lassa, Ebola, Marburg and Crimea-Congo are the main suspects, but Dengue fever is the most common and is the only one that does not presently occur in Africa, being confined to South-East Asia, South America and the western Pacific. In the majority of cases, Dengue will cause a short-lived feverish illness with a rash. However, in a proportion, particularly with a second infection, the haemorrhagic variant of Dengue may arise. This is where part of the horror of these conditions arises: the blood ceases to clot, and death is by failure of organs in which massive bleeding may occur. Dengue is transmitted by mosquitoes, but all the others are so potentially dangerous and transmissible that specialist units have to be maintained on stand-by to nurse confirmed victims. There are two methods of doing so: so-called Trexler beds, which are thick polythene cages with controlled entry and exit ports and special reduced pressure ventilation to reduce the possibility of infection through aerosols, and nursing the patient while wearing specialised body suits.

Suppose you have returned from Nigeria, where you have been working on a relief project clearing bush in a rural area for a refugee camp; you were much troubled by ubiquitous rats during your work. You begin to feel unwell with a high temperature and something of a backache. You consult a doctor. Most physicians would consider malaria as a likely diagnosis at this juncture; however, a simple blood test suggests it is not so. At this moment, loud alarm bells should be ringing in the doctor's ears; in fact, this does not always happen and not every case of VHF is picked up at this moment, with potentially disastrous consequences. However, on this occasion the wide-awake doctor calls up his local infectious diseases colleague for advice, and a well-rehearsed protocol swings into action.

All further tests on your blood are suspended; it is potentially infectious. A specialist team of volunteer ambulance men, wearing protective gear, is activated to transfer the patient to the specialist unit. There are two in Britain: Coppett's Wood, North London and Newcastle. Placed in isolation, the only contact the patient has with friends and relatives is via an intercom. A trained specialist will take one further blood sample and send it in secure packaging by courier to the reference laboratories at Colindale and Porton Down, where they have facilities to confirm the diagnosis.

In the cases where the diagnosis is confirmed, there is a prolonged stay in the big plastic bubble until either recovery or death ensues. And this death is unpleasant; haemorrhage can occur from any part of the body including the eyes and nose. It is blood in the lungs that actually causes the final event. I could have included the VHFs in the 'untreatable infections' category, but there is some suggestion that the antiviral drug ribavirin may reduce mortality. Nor is the disease exclusively fatal; a nurse contracted Lassa following a case in Britain and was only found to have it in subsequent blood tests. Furthermore, when people living in areas where Ebola is endemic have their blood tested, a significant number have antibodies to the virus implying non-fatal infection.

While these diseases may seem exotic to some in the West, a few are not even that rare: 12 million people are believed to be infected with leishmaniasis, 18 million with Chagas' Disease. However, these strange infections do illustrate a point. Almost all of the diseases I have mentioned in this chapter are not confined simply to human infection. Livestock are more severely affected by screw-worm than humans; *Leishmania* infects dogs, in addition to a number of other animals; opossums and possibly goats act as reservoirs for South American trypanosomiasis. Monkeys carry Marburg and Dengue; ostrich ticks Crimea–Congo; rats Lassa; gorillas and other primates probably carry Ebola. The close, domestic approximation of man and animal is a relatively recent phenomenon in evolutionary terms. The change in human behaviour from nomadic hunter–gatherer to settled agrarian or herdsman represented a significant step towards our civilisation. Thus, acquiring infections from domestic animals or livestock is one of the prices we have had to pay for becoming 'advanced'. Had we acquired the infections earlier in our evolutionary history, we may have developed a greater degree of resistance to them. This point is clearly illustrated by the different forms of skin leishmaniasis contracted by native South Americans and visiting workers. Infection with the same bug – *Leishmania mexicana* – causes transient, mild infections in the resident Amerindians. By contrast, incoming forestry workers may develop disfiguring and mutilating infections of the nose and mouth. Loa loa demonstrates the same phenomenon: visitors who have never previously encountered the parasite will suffer far more serious infections than the indigenous population.

These horrible rarities are far from being the only infectious diseases that man has acquired from animals; one of the greatest killers of all, TB, is believed to have mutated from a similar organism found in cows. It appeared in humans at about the time we began to keep cattle in barns and sheds near or in our houses. We share our world with many types of life, and the vast majority of life forms pose no threat to us. However, every time we change our behaviour we expose ourselves to new types of infection from new sources. This may be from herding animals or wholesale butchering of wild animals in once remote rainforests. Every time we turn a new corner, we encounter a new Quiet Killer, or awaken a sleeping one. Each of the infections we have discussed in this chapter may be unpleasant and frightening, but at least all are treatable. In the next chapter, we will examine a number of illnesses where, as yet, we do not have that luxury.

NINE

Persistent and Invasive
Untreatable infections

Is there such a thing as an infectious disease which cannot be treated? Are there any diseases that mean absolutely certain death? If so, is that problem getting worse? The answer to all of these questions is yes. You could divide 'untreatable' infectious diseases into a number of categories. The first group would comprise infections for which we have not yet been able to find a decent treatment, and may never do so. The second group might contain those infections which we though we had licked, but are coming back. These will be discussed later.

So, which infectious diseases are 'untreatable?' In a sense, no disease is. Even if doctors cannot cure a disease, something can usually be offered to relieve unpleasant symptoms. Take cryptosporidiosis. This is caused by a parasite, *Cryptosporidium parvum*. The condition it leads to is profound, watery diarrhoea, which may be as prolific in its output as in cholera. There is no treatment for cryptosporidiosis that will reliably cure the disease. Like most illnesses that cause diarrhoea, the major hazard is a degree of dehydration and salt loss that will cause kidney failure and death. If salt and water losses are replaced, most healthy people will spontaneously eliminate the infection. This may have to happen in hospital, but usually the disease is not fatal.

Cryptosporidium parvum is a remarkable organism in several respects. First, by the standards of the protozoa, the group to which it belongs, it is tiny. This makes it difficult to filter from drinking water supplies like reservoirs. It slips into swimming pools from infected individuals and is potentially very highly infectious. There is one well-documented case where every single person who swam in a particular pool became infected with the parasite. The problem arises in patients with damaged immunity, such as HIV/AIDS, when the infection may be prolonged and fatal.

Cryptosporidium parvum is by no means the only Quiet Killer for which there is no effective treatment. Tropical spastic paraparesis is a peculiarly unpleasant paralytic consequence of infection with a virus called HTLV-1 (Human T-lymphotrophic Virus type-1). It shows both a geographical and a genetic predilection for people from the Caribbean, Japan and Papua New Guinea. HTLV-1 appears to be transmitted sexually and through blood and breast milk. It may also transmit from mother to child in the womb. It has other unpleasant consequences also: the virus seems to trigger certain kinds of cancer, including a condition called adult T-cell leukaemia. Some scientists believe that drugs effective against HIV may be beneficial, but there is really very little evidence to date. A combination of interferon alpha and the HIV drug AZT has been reported to be effective in treating patients with the leukaemia. A muscle relaxant called danazol, and Vitamin C may provide temporary relief for patients with tropical spastic paraparesis. Vaccines are being developed, and screening of mothers to advise them not to breastfeed is carried out in places where there is a high incidence. However, I am afraid if you live in an area of high incidence and have genetic susceptibility then there is very little that can be done.

*   *   *

Like HTLV-1, nvCJD is an illness which requires both a genetically susceptible host and exposure to the agent. What is most strange about nvCJD – new variant Creutzfeldt-Jakob Disease – is not so much that it is virtually untreatable, nor that it is an apparently 'new' disease caused by a totally different agent to the other Quiet Killers, but what was done in its name. An entire industry – the raising of beef in Britain – was almost destroyed on the basis of scientific advice, and predictions of the disease's eventual spread have proven wildly inaccurate.

New variant CJD is an extremely unpleasant condition. It tends to afflict people of a lower age and has a shorter incubation period than its cousins, the other so-called transmissible spongiform encephalopathies. The median age of onset is a tragic 28. The early symptoms are memory loss, mood changes, hallucinations, loss of judgement, and posture and balance disturbance, progressing inexorably to painful muscle spasms, stupor, coma and death. Its victims take a little over a year to die.

BSE, the cattle variant of the disease, was an apparently new illness, first diagnosed in the United Kingdom in November 1986. Many will recall the extraordinary press footage of cows lurching and staggering wildly like punch-drunk prize-fighters. Over the next few years, the epidemic spread and affected just about the entire country. Other European nations were affected, even those which subsequently banned the import of British beef and cattle. The outbreak reached its peak in 1992, when 36,680 cases were confirmed, and since then has shown a steady decline.

At this point, I should make it quite clear that I have had to make a judgement about the causation of BSE and nvCJD. Multiple hypotheses have been advanced, including organophosphate poisoning, heavy metals, viruses and incomplete bacteria called *Mycoplasma*. The prion hypothesis, advanced by Stanley Prusiner, appears to me to be far and away the most convincing. I make no apology for rejecting any competing theory for the purposes of this book. My object is to demonstrate the extraordinary diversity and cunning of infectious diseases among our species, not to rehearse complex and partisan scientific debates.

Every other Quiet Killer that we have encountered is made up of essentially the same components. Viruses, bacteria, parasites and fungi all rely on the basic genetic code of either DNA or RNA or both for their structure and transmission. The agents causing BSE, and its relations Kuru, Gerstmann-Sträussler, scrapie, mink encephalopathy, chronic wasting disease of deer and Creutzfeldt-Jakob Disease, are composed of no such material. They are, as far as we know, entirely different in the manner in which they cause disease. They do this by triggering a critical change in the conformation of proteins within nerve tissue. Instead of being set out in orderly sheets of structured material, the proteins are laid down in tangled, matted masses that disrupt normal neurochemical transmission. It is a little like a complex knitted garment where a single dropped stitch can cause the whole to unravel. The agents of these illnesses seem to be simply proteins themselves, with no known genes of their own. They are called prions.

These proteins are transmissible. A number of people were tragically infected with a similar illness during treatments with human pituitary extracts as growth stimulators. In humans, it would seem that, as in HTLV-1, the correct conformation of genetic elements is required to proceed from simple exposure to disease. The number of people who carry the structure of genes that makes them susceptible to nvCJD is potentially enormous. The best available evidence was that the agent was carried in beef products, and in tiny quantities. It seemed to have leaped over the species barrier – in fact, for this reason, many scientists prefer the term 'species hurdle'. The current hypothesis is that it did so by being passed back through cattle in feedstuffs made of recovered protein, including recovered meat from cattle themselves and from sheep. Sheep harbour a related condition called scrapie. The cattle were unwitting cannibals and carnivores, in fact.

Beef products are ubiquitous; they are a basic constituent of many gelatine-based foodstuffs, including the most unlikely substances such as children's sweets. Prion proteins are not destroyed by cooking, nor even by routine sterilisation of surgical instruments. Therefore, a huge number of potentially susceptible individuals had been exposed. This explains the extraordinary lengths that the British government and others went to in their attempts to eradicate BSE from the cattle herd.

There are a number of problems with interpreting and acting upon this apparently straightforward hypothesis. Transmissible spongiform encephalopathies may have a very long incubation period. Kuru is a related disease that afflicts societies that eat human flesh – cannibals, bluntly. The incubation period in kuru may be as long as thirty or forty years. Its duration appears to be related to the natural lifespan of the victim. In cows, BSE has an average

174

incubation period of 5.2 years. It is much longer in humans, with our three-score and ten life expectancy. In other words, there was likely to be a lag before we started to see large numbers of people with BSE, or more accurately its human equivalent, new variant CJD. It was therefore very difficult to predict what the likely future number of affected cases might be.

The incidence of CJD is monitored in the United Kingdom by the national CJD surveillance unit based at the Western General Hospital in Edinburgh, Scotland. At the time of writing, the unit has had referred 2,043 possible cases. The total number of deaths is 1,105. You might think this was reasonable grounds for defining an epidemic. However, the figures conceal a number of caveats. First, the diagnosis has not been confirmed in all cases. It is not easy to diagnose, and referrals include patients with peculiar neurological conditions in whom no other diagnosis has been made. The diagnosis can presently only really be made by examination of biopsied tissue. Other tests such as MRI scans, electroencephalograms recording abnormal electrical activity in the brain, and examination of spinal fluid may be suggestive but not diagnostic. Brain biopsy is a risky procedure in life, and is usually only conducted at post-mortem. Tissue from potentially affected patients has to be handled with extreme care as it may be infectious. The unit monitors not only new variant CJD (nvCJD), but also the sporadic, familial and pituitary extract forms of the disease, all of which occurred before the BSE crisis. It also monitors related conditions such as Gerstmann-Sträussler. New variant CJD has been confirmed in 109 people who have died. There are 6 living with a probable diagnosis. A further 44 died with probable nvCJD, with the diagnosis unconfirmed. The peak year was 2000, when 28 died. The number of cases has declined since, with 20, 17, 18, 9 and 5 in the succeeding years until 2005. There have been a further 6 in France, 2 in Canada and 1 each in Ireland, Italy and the United States. You might argue that the government's ban on beef older than three years entering the food chain has been successful. However, it does bring into question those predictions about hospices in every town.

New variant CJD is tragically among the untreatable infections. We simply know too little about prions to be able to interfere in their life cycles (if, indeed, they can be said to be alive) in the way that we can with other organisms. Prions have no cell walls; no growing chains of DNA; no paths of vitamin synthesis – in short, none of the targets which make the other Quiet Killers susceptible. There has been some progress in the development of a sieve to extract the agent from blood transfusions. A drug called pentosan polysulphate (PPS) may or may not work. The problem with diseases like nvCJD is that the numbers afflicted and treated are so tiny.

*   *   *

Infections may, of course, become untreatable by acquiring resistance to antibiotics. There are a number of means by which the Quiet Killers can do this. Some of the actual 'how' of resistance has been discussed in the introduction. Here, I examine the 'why' of antibiotic resistance, and then investigate how – if at all – they actually cause untreatable disease.

The most commonly held view of how antibiotic resistance arose is that the doctors are at fault; we squandered our advantage over infections by wantonly prescribing antibiotics to patients just to be shot of them. Even if this were wholly true, I speak from experience when I say that the expectation of a demanding patient is as important in this transaction as the weary resignation of the doctor. Whatever the case, the tide in many countries has turned in this respect. In Britain, many hospitals are appointing specialist pharmacists who deal solely with prescriptions relating to infection; in one instance, a pharmacist managed to save her employers more than her entire annual salary by analysing and restricting the inappropriate issuing of drugs.

Part of the problem is that it is very difficult to obtain good hard evidence for making decisions. Take middle ear infections in children. These are common and may lead to deafness and learning difficulties if they recur. The evidence is that antibiotics do not necessarily prevent recurrence; at best, they reduce both the risk of dangerous complications, such as spreading local infections, and the duration of painful symptoms, by three days. Naturally, the risk of infection with resistant organisms is increased by exposure to drugs. Some doctors feel that antibiotic-prescribing is therefore not appropriate; others take the opposite view. Which is right?

In some parts of the world, antibiotics may be obtained over the counter without a prescription. I recall being amazed at my possible choices when I bought some antibiotics in Thailand; I had fallen off a rented motor scooter and developed an infected thumb. Even in a small provincial pharmacy, I could have had just about any oral medication, even some that would be on restricted lists in most British hospitals. For this reason, rates of resistance vary hugely throughout the world. Typhoid, for instance, has become resistant to the very useful antibiotic ciprofloxacin in many parts of Asia. This is true of other bacteria also: in southern Europe, over 30 per cent of *Pseudomonas aeruginosa* – a cause of pneumonia in hospitals, among other things – is resistant to ciprofloxacin, while in northern Europe, the figure is closer to 7 per cent.

Lax prescribing and poor restriction of antibiotics to the public is only part of the problem. Many will know that antibiotics are not solely used by the medical profession. Within agriculture, they have been used widely and in industrial quantities. Antibiotics are used in animals to treat and to prevent infections. They are also used extensively in low doses to promote growth by increasing weight gain and improving feed utilisation. Take, for instance, avoparcin. It was used from the 1970s to the 1990s in Europe as a growth promoter in chickens, pigs, calves, beef and dairy cattle. It is also approved for preventing the unpleasant gut-killing necrotic enteritis (caused by the gas gangrene bacterium *Clostridium perfringens*) in broiler chickens. It was used in massive quantities which dwarfed human usage. For example, in Denmark, 24,000kg of avoparcin was used annually in animals in 1994, compared with 24kg of equivalent antibiotics in humans; in Austria, corresponding figures were 20,000kg versus 66kg. Avoparcin belongs to the same group of drugs as vancomycin and teicoplanin; the primary use for these drugs in humans is for MRSA and *Enterococcus* infections. These antibiotics have been regarded as the last hope in patients with these infections.

177

What happened next illustrates the phenomenal capacity of the Quiet Killers to adapt in response to challenge from human intervention. You might have thought that an antibiotic given primarily to farm animals – and one that is different to that used in humans – would have simply caused avoparcin-resistant bacteria to emerge in those animals alone. However, not long after avoparcin was widely introduced, *Enterococci* with resistance to the related antibiotics vancomycin and teicoplanin began to appear in humans. The most convincing early link occurred in a farm worker with a fracture that became infected with VRE (Vancomycin-Resistant *Enterococcus*). He had been exposed to avoparcin in his working life. Gradually, it became clear that VRE was slipping into the food chain. It was rarely found in communities where avoparcin had not been used, and commonly so where it had. In the United States, where avoparcin was never licensed for use in animals, where VRE arose it did so from single hospital sources, originating in New York and leaping from hospital to hospital. In avoparcin-using countries, VRE was ubiquitous in animals and their food products; in the Netherlands, in 1998, 79 per cent of poultry products contained VRE. It began to appear in the intestines of humans who had been given no antibiotics: VRE was found in the bowel of 2 per cent to 17 per cent of the general community in countries including the United Kingdom, the Netherlands, Germany and Belgium. For vancomycin resistance to emerge, a complex series of genetic events has to occur in the bacterium, not just a simple single change. This made it highly likely that VRE was being eaten with animal products, rather than mutating spontaneously in the human body. The most clinching piece of evidence came from the fact that different mutations occur in VRE in different animals. Pig VRE is genetically different from poultry VRE. In people who ate pig meat, pig VRE appeared; in communities who eschewed the pig, chicken VRE took its place.

Enterococci are exceptionally good at transmitting this variety of resistance among one another and to related species. In the laboratory, this property has even been spread to *Staphylococcus aureus*, giving rise to the worrisome prospect of MRSA that is highly resistant to vancomycin. *Enterococci* are perfectly capable of causing disease in otherwise sick people. However, *Staphylococcus aureus* is altogether a more unpleasant bacterium, capable of causing death and severe illness in healthy young people.

At the time of writing, it is probably this bug – or 'superbug' – which is causing more terror and anxiety than any other apart from bird flu. It seems only a moment ago that the newspapers were fretting about the 'flesh-eating virus' (actually not caused by a virus at all) necrotising fasciitis. As is always the case with these panics, they quickly move on, being immediately replaced by something else; and that something else is the scourge called MRSA.

So just how dangerous is the infection? Any infectious agent – be it a virus, a bacterium like *Staphylococcus aureus*, or a parasite like malaria – depends on two basic principles to cause disease. One is the resilience of the victim. The other is the virulence of the bug itself, the weapons that it carries. *Staphylococcus aureus*, whether MRSA or not, has a pretty impressive armoury. It has enzymes to liquefy fat, sinew and bone. It produces a poison that will prostrate you with diarrhoea and vomiting in hours. It can generate a toxin that makes its victim's skin simply drop off, especially if that victim is a baby; this is the so-called scalded skin syndrome.

However, these big guns are no good to the germ unless it can get into you somehow and avoid being eaten by your immune system. You and I can live with MRSA on our skin; many of us do so without realising it. But if it gets into the blood, you're in trouble. The simplest route of entry is injection, particularly if you're a drug user who's not too fussy about their works. I've helplessly watched several foolish young people die with their heart valves shredded by MRSA. In hospitals, it can skulk into the blood of the elderly after an operation, settling especially on the bones. MRSA in the blood gives you a 30 per cent chance of survival, about the same rate as smallpox before Jenner's vaccine came along.

We have been here before with this bug. It has been around since about 1961. Ten jumbo jets crashing every year is equivalent to the annual MRSA death toll. Worry seems queasily feeble in the face of such carnage. Shouldn't we panic?

Some already are. I know of one elderly gentleman who isolated himself in his own home for six weeks because he had MRSA. It was living harmlessly on the skin in his armpit. I know of another case where an MRSA-colonised mother was told to stop breastfeeding her baby – by a midwife, as it happens, who should have known better.

You may realise that, although unfortunate, neither of these scenarios is common. Those ten jumbo jetsful are hotly disputed figures. There's an obvious difference between dying with MRSA and merely having MRSA; the less obvious concern is deciding how much MRSA contributes to any given death. Compared to the mortality from heart disease, say, MRSA is a spear-carrier.

There is a more dangerous variant of *S. aureus*, containing a toxin called Panton-Valentine leukocidin, which is becoming more common. Apart from causing boils, this poison kills young, healthy people with a peculiarly vicious pneumonia. In Britain, it occurs in about 2 per cent of the MRSA cases we are currently seeing in out-of-hospital, community infections. In some American studies, the figure is closer to 20 per cent. Now *that* is worrying.

The real cause for anxiety about MRSA, though, is what it tells us about the ability of all bacteria to scoff at our clever new antibiotics. It is far from being alone. Bacteria are astonishingly deft at acquiring resistance and transmitting it to one another. This is discussed elsewhere, but it is clear that a small number of bugs are becoming effectively untreatable. There is, nonetheless, some hope for the future and we will discuss this in the final chapter.

There is, of course, another reason why an infectious disease may be untreatable, and that is where the political will or the finance is simply not present. So it is in much of the world with respect to HIV. There is even one state where the scientifically incontrovertible link between HIV and AIDS is officially denied, although this position is reportedly softening. I am conscious that the association between poverty, the state of the developing nations and infectious diseases has become something of a mantra in this book. In the words of South African President Thabo Mbeki himself: 'The world's biggest killer and the greatest cause of ill-health and suffering across the globe is listed almost at the end of the International Classification of Diseases. It is given the code Z59.5 – extreme poverty.' I propose to offer a variation on the theme. We have become familiar with a demand from some quarters that cheap anti-HIV medication be made available for developing countries. However, well-meaning efforts to secure a supply of affordable HIV medication for the Third World may make matters far, far worse, and may even lead to untreatable infection in both the poorer and the western nations.

As we have seen in other chapters, viruses are more prone to mutation than other, more complex life forms. Mutation is more likely to arise where there is a need for it to do so; or at least a mutation with some competitive advantage is more likely to reproduce in this new environment where there is evolutionary pressure to do so. A drug active against a virus may provide precisely this necessary evolutionary pressure. In other words, viruses can mutate to develop resistance against drugs, and the presence of the drugs encourages such resistance to develop. We now know that to suppress mutations causing resistance to HIV we need to use combinations of drugs, usually three. Ensuring that mutations do not arise is an extremely demanding task, especially in the early days of treatment. One of the key tasks of any physician treating HIV is to impress upon patients the absolute necessity not to miss any medication. During the early days, the quantity of virus in the blood is carefully measured. A rise or inadequate fall in the so-called 'viral load' despite effective drugs is a cause for concern. There are several reasons why this vital early treatment might not be taken as completely as it should. Patients may find the tablets unbearable due to side effects. Additionally, remembering to take the tablets is not as easy as you might think. Some medication requires special storage, or must be taken with food, or on an empty stomach. The eventual result may be failure not only of treatment, but the virus may also acquire resistance to some or all of the drugs.

Monitoring therapy is expensive and complex. The back-up is skilled and costly; it involves the interpretation of single changes in the virus's genetic code. There is a further technical difficulty in that the sample you collect from your patient will contain multiple versions of the virus, some with the resistant mutations and some without. If the patient stops taking the medication, the resistant virus may apparently temporarily 'disappear' as the mutant no longer has the selection advantage provided by the presence of the drug. It is almost a matter of chance whether you examine the resistant version or the original, so-called 'wild' type. Once the virus has acquired resistance, it may be transmitted to a new victim in its resistant form. Eventually, if a sufficient number of resistant mutations arise, the virus becomes untreatable.

Supposing, then, cheap HIV drugs are supplied to countries that do not have the sophisticated facilities required to monitor the disease. The potential consequence is widespread resistance, which may ultimately transmit. The advances made in HIV treatment over recent years may be lost.

This may seem unfair, and a counsel of despair. There is, though, no shortage of examples of infectious diseases which have become harder to treat through inconsistent issuing of antibiotics. The most telling example is TB. This condition, much like HIV but on a shorter time-scale, requires persistent and reliable treatment. HIV treatment (currently) needs to be continued indefinitely. TB requires a minimum period of six months, but only if the treatment is taken correctly. Without constant and regular doses of the drugs, the bacterium rapidly acquires resistance.

What is most depressing is the litany of terrible reasons why TB drugs may not be taken reliably in developing countries. People cannot afford the drugs, so they stop taking them. They need money, so they sell them on. The wrong drugs are prescribed. People feel better after a couple of weeks' treatment, and there is not an adequate health system to pursue the issue. Most distressingly of all, there is a thriving market in fake, chalk tablets packaged to look like the real thing. For this reason, in one study in Nigeria, TB had a cure rate of 10 per cent. Only about half of the tablets prescribed were correct, for the range of reasons listed above. This compares to a cure rate of 90 per cent in the developed world. The chances in

Nigeria of the partly treated 90 per cent harbouring resistant TB is high indeed. Multi-resistant TB is difficult, if not impossible, to treat. Supposing the same were to be repeated in HIV – only 10 per cent correctly treated, with the remaining 90 per cent acquiring resistance?

We have already seen multi-resistant TB in Britain and the United States, as well as in Africa and in prisons in Russia. It would be a tragedy if the victories we have achieved over HIV medication were to be squandered through the same error, indiscriminate prescribing, that has put us on the back foot with so many of the other Quiet Killers.

*   *   *

It could have been so very much worse, and we should thank our lucky stars for the lessons it has taught us. Above all, both luck and the weather played a major part. Severe acute respiratory syndrome (SARS) was first drawn to widespread attention by a doctor working in Vietnam for the World Health Organization called Dr Carlo Urbani.

This diligent and concerned physician was anxious about the unexplained illness of his patient, an American businessman called Johnny Cheng. Over a matter of four days in March 2003, Cheng had declined from being a fit middle-aged man to near death. He was having difficulty breathing, had a high fever and a rasping cough, and his lungs were filling up with fluid. None of the treatments Urbani tried seemed to make any difference. He contacted his employers at the WHO, concerned that he was witnessing some new type of infection. He was most worried that it could be the first sign of a new flu epidemic.

Urbani's anxiety was more justified than even he could have imagined. The illness was rapidly claiming other victims throughout the Hanoi hospital. Cheng, a nurse and another doctor soon died. Then, Urbani himself became ill. Tragically, the man who had first alerted us to this new disease joined the long list of physicians like Ricketts whose own lives have been claimed by the diseases which they studied or treated.

Cheng was known to have travelled through Guangdong Province, along the border with Hong Kong, before he flew to Vietnam. There had been rumours of disease circulating in that area. The WHO contacted the Chinese authorities, who, true to their traditionally secretive nature, delayed in responding but did finally admit that there had been 40 cases of an unexplained illness. They said that the outbreak was under control, and that although they had not identified a cause they had eliminated a number of diseases from their list of suspects, such as Ebola, anthrax and Lassa fever.

Alarm bells began to ring when two cases were reported in Hong Kong. The legacies of Britain's last great crown colony include extremely dense population and rapid international communications across the globe. The WHO was deeply concerned; if this was another flu outbreak, it could spread at the speed of a jet aircraft across the world and millions could die. Urgent action needed to be taken. It was decided to break open the War Plan.

The War Plan is a detailed document with instructions for action in the event of a developing world pandemic. It had been hoped never to have to open it, but now the risks of allowing this disease to transmit across the globe were just too great. Contained within the document is a dire warning of what might happen if such action were to fail: economic and social collapse might follow.

The first step, it was generally agreed, was to identify the cause. Specimens were collected from the Hanoi victims. The task of hunting the cause was given to Dr Klaus Stohr, because he was the WHO's influenza expert. Until that moment, most believed that flu was the likely cause. It was with mixed relief and panic that the team learned that the initial tests for flu were negative. They were also negative for the viral haemorrhagic fevers, for pulmonary hantavirus, and for every other rarity anyone could think of. The team were temporarily stumped.

Meanwhile, the outbreak was gathering pace. There had been twenty-five new cases in Hong Kong and twenty-six in Vietnam. From Toronto, Canada came the terrifying news that a mother and son who had travelled to Hong Kong had fallen ill and died with similar symptoms. Four further members of the same family came down with the illness; and then Pat Tamlin, a nurse on the intensive care unit of the same Toronto hospital, fell ill with what she described as 'the worst illness I had ever had'. Fortunately, she survived, but a distant outbreak from the probable epicentre, with medical personnel affected, was just too much. On 15 March 2003, a panicked WHO announced 'World Wide Alert', and gave the illness, which has a mortality somewhere between 1 in 10 and 1 in 25, its name – SARS. They issued instructions for hospitals throughout the world, including how to isolate victims and what protective clothing to wear.

The results were astonishing. Within twenty-four hours, it became clear that this was already a worldwide phenomenon. There were reported cases in South-East Asia, the Pacific, and even Germany. Most seemed to have a connection with Hong Kong, which by now had more than 100 reported cases.

Stohr decided to call in the world's experts. There were eleven different units summoned to the team, including the Centers for Disease Control in America, the Institut Pasteur in France and Britain's Colindale Laboratory. All agreed to collaborate, a remarkable achievement given the traditional rivalry between academic institutions.

With an amazing stroke of luck, Dr Thomas Tsang, of the Chinese University and Government Virus Unit in Hong Kong, managed to find the source, or index patient, for the Hong Kong outbreak. Tsang had, by diligent and dogged analysis, found a link between eight of the victims. Johnny Cheng, the Hanoi victim; an air hostess who had been the first case in Singapore; and the mother who had taken the disease to Toronto – all had something in common. They had all stayed at the same hotel, called the Metropole. The importance of this discovery cannot be overestimated. Once you know how an outbreak arose, you can deduce how it transmits and then interrupt that transmission. Tsang was even able to find the very first Hong Kong SARS victim. His name was Liu Jianlun, and he was a doctor from China.

These pieces of information yielded far more than seems initially obvious. The rumours of a nasty new illness in Guangdong were confirmed; by now, it had spread to four other provinces. Transmission to medical staff was also, tragically, confirmed. But what conclusion would you draw from the fact that many of these first victims had stayed on the same floor of the Metropole hotel? Surprisingly, it told the WHO investigators that SARS was really not that infectious. Had the virus been as readily transmissible as chickenpox, say, or smallpox, then there would have been victims on every floor of the hotel, and other hotels, offices and homes besides. It would have been almost impossible to trace the index patient among such random, everyday casual contacts. But SARS seemed to require much closer physical encounters, such as perhaps touching a doorknob or lift-button that a patient incubating SARS had just touched.

This may seem to be a piece of evidence of merely academic interest. There is, however, a far more important conclusion to be drawn. If the disease were not particularly easy to transmit, then straightforward, simple and not especially radical methods of isolation should be adequate to control it. No international airport closures, no school shutdowns, no martial law would be necessary.

The authorities were naturally very keen to identify some telltale sign that might help to diagnose possible cases. Pat Tamlin, the Canadian nurse who had contracted SARS from a patient and survived, provides the major clue to the key disease indicator in her description of her symptoms: 'I was working one night in Intensive Care when I noticed I was unusually warm. So I happened to take my temperature and it was 38.7°C which is significantly high. And I knew that I was getting more ill as time went on.' Of course, high fevers may be a sign of many different illnesses. But as a means of screening large numbers for a rare illness, it's hard to beat.

Based on this kind of evidence – high fever during incubation – an unprecedented step was taken in many parts of the world. Arrivals at airports would be screened by thermal imaging cameras; in Singapore, this meant that even cabinet members and the Prime Minister himself routinely had their temperatures measured on arrival for work.

On 21 March, the riddle of SARS was solved, when the team from Hong Kong dramatically announced that they had identified the virus. Their discovery had come about from a combination of shrewd hunches, technical dexterity and extreme luck. Basically, they had randomly tested for DNA and RNA to every known virus – a process called random primer sampling – in the hope that something would come up. The sheer serendipity of their discovery is not really conveyed by these simple words. It is a little like trying to identify a foreign language by using only anagrams. Nevertheless, they pulled it off and named the virus as belonging to the coronavirus group. You and I will have almost certainly encountered these relatively benign beasts in our lifetimes; they cause an illness indistinguishable from the common cold. This one, though, had gone rogue.

What do I mean by that? Rogue sharks are those that have developed a 'taste' for human flesh, and neglect their usual diet of seals, turtles and fish in our favour. This is precisely what happened to the SARS virus. Dietary habits in parts of China are, by western standards, remarkably inclusive. This means that human contact with wild animal species – in husbandry, hunting, butchery and consumption – is far closer than in the more squeamish culture of the West. Viruses are transmitted from animals to humans in these circumstances all the time. The vast majority are incapable of attaching to receptors on our cells; they have evolved to attach to the receptors of their usual hosts. Where contact is repeated and systematic, then the chances of a mutation that can leap the species hurdle is far more likely. The virus goes 'rogue'; its craving for the flesh of the human becomes insatiable. There is no effective treatment for the coronavirus. Various drugs have been tried; the best we can hope for is to keep the patient alive until they recover spontaneously.

The identification of the actual virus, although vital, played only a small part in the containment of this incurable illness. The containment of Nipah virus, the unpleasant new scourge spread from pigs in Malaysia, will be discussed in Chapter Ten. That outbreak was controlled by means that would have been understood by John Snow, the anaesthetist who founded the rudiments of public health medicine 170 years ago. So it was with SARS. It is salutary that the first affected country to be declared free of SARS was probably the poorest – Vietnam. The worst affected country – China – reflects a different paradigm for infection control. Secretive, dogmatic and paranoid, the Chinese responded by concealment and subsequently denying the full extent of the problem. They paid the price, however. Their final case load was way in excess of their original figures; in the hundreds rather than tens. The truth may never be known, but figures in the order of 400 are widely acknowledged, with a mortality of about 10 per cent. The official figures are these: during November 2002 to July 2003, a total of 8,098 probable cases of SARS were reported to the WHO from 29 countries, including 29 cases from the United States; 774 SARS-related deaths (case-fatality rate: 9.6 per cent) were reported, none of which occurred in the United States. Reporting of cases ended in July 2003.

There was an element of luck in the SARS story; the weather also played a part. The disease arose in China and the Far East shortly before spring in the northern hemisphere. By April in Europe, the winter is usually a memory; sometimes, the weather in March is warm enough to take many out into the parks and open spaces. So it was in that spring of 2003. On 23 March, two days after the virus was identified and while the epidemic was still at its peak, the temperature in Central London rose to 20.0°C. The mean temperature for March was 2.0°C above the benchmark 1961–90 mean, which is in the 'exceptionally above average' category. Rainfall was sparce and sunshine plentiful; in fact, the sunniest March on record. In short, it was an exceptionally warm, dry spring. SARS seemed to need contact in enclosed spaces like lobbies and lifts, and nobody in Europe was spending much time indoors during that period. The outcome might have been very different if the disease had arisen in China in early December; or even if the weather in Europe had been cold and miserable, much as it was in Toronto. Our victory over SARS in Europe may have been, like the defeat of Napoleon and Hitler in Russia, more climatic than tactical.

Paradoxically, global warming may have contained this new disease. Perhaps next time we will not be so fortunate.

Not every infectious illness is given a formal diagnosis, even in modern hospitals. Many find this surprising. So a kind of perverted and cruel luck applied with SARS. Urbani worked for the World Health Organization and was primed to look for influenza; indeed, that's one of the reasons he was so concerned about Johnny Cheng. Would every physician have been as diligent in the same circumstances? Would every doctor have taken the vital step of contacting the WHO as early as Urbani did? There is no doubt that this early alert made a huge difference. Such lessons as these that we have learned from SARS will prove invaluable in the event of any flu pandemic, or indeed any other incurable infection. This thought leads us naturally into our next chapter and some of the newer diseases which are troubling us.

TEN

New Scourges and Resurgent Diseases

Recent years have seen the emergence of several 'new' infections in man, notably HIV. But there are others – Hendra and Nipah virus, and the potential new scourge of West Nile Fever. Are these really new? Why are they troubling us now?

How do you know that you have a new disease? The symptoms and signs of many illnesses are similar, whatever the cause; it takes a skilled doctor to distinguish between even a simple sore throat caused by a virus and one caused by bacteria without lab tests. This explains why doctors sometimes get it wrong, and why so many prescriptions for antibiotics have been issued for viral sore throats when they don't work. The same is true of most of the Quiet Killers. Pneumonia, for example, may cause identical symptoms whether caused by *Streptococcus pneumoniae* or any other of the huge number of bugs that can infect the lungs. It is only recently, since science has been able to differentiate, that we have made the distinction. The discrimination is obviously important, to ensure that the doctor is giving the right treatment. It may be that the definition of any disease as 'new' is potentially flawed. We may have encountered it before, but simply failed to recognise it. Conversely to the way in which the Bloody Flux vanished as a diagnosis when the true causes of blood-stained diarrhoea were established, improved technology has meant that the origins of some of the 'newer' Quiet Killers can be given a precise name.

The first step to defining a new disease is, therefore, to recognise the emergence of a fresh pattern. Two of the classic patterns are totally new symptoms, never before encountered, and a cluster of conventional illnesses in a previously unaffected population. Let us consider the latter, more common, situation first. Many people who are not doctors would be surprised by the number of people who are unwell, admitted to hospital even, and yet are never given a formal diagnosis. Even in severe brain infections, the rate of isolation of the true cause rarely exceeds 50 per cent. The patient may leave hospital, should they recover, with the imprecise label of 'meningitis' or 'encephalitis'. Thus, unless there is some other feature to cause concern, the threshold for a doctor believing that they are dealing with a new disease may actually be quite high.

There are many perfectly valid reasons for this imprecision. Many family or emergency doctors presented with someone with possible meningitis would prefer to treat them with antibiotics on the basis of suspicion, in the hope of saving the patient's life. This will inevitably reduce the diagnostic yield, because it then may not be possible to grow the causative bug in the laboratory, damaged as it is by the drugs. The technology available to diagnose many diseases is imperfect; many of the Quiet Killers are capricious when encouraged to reveal themselves in the laboratory, and simply refuse to do so. Nor are all diagnostic facilities available in every laboratory. Smaller institutions will generally confine themselves to identifying the more common and life-threatening conditions, not being able to afford the more expensive equipment sometimes required to detect more esoteric infections. Additionally, not all laboratories use the same equipment or techniques, which introduces unreliable results; and then, of course, there is human error.

Of course, not all cases of a new disease will present to the same doctor or even in the same country. Early alarm bells ringing therefore depends on efficient communication. However, even in countries with efficient communications, modern facilities and well-trained doctors, detection of a new disease can go badly wrong.

Malaysia is just such a country. The facilities in Kuala Lumpur compared favourably with Britain's NHS, of which we used to be so proud. In 1998–9, Malaysian doctors were alarmed to notice a sudden increase in patients suffering from encephalitis. This outbreak had high death rates and occurred in a small community in Tambun, in the province of Perak. The disease spread southwards. Within four to six months, several other communities near or around Seremban, a city about 300km from Tambun, were affected. By April 1999, at least 85 deaths were reported in Seremban; 15 were recorded in Tambun. The illness also spread to Singapore. In March 1999, four abattoir personnel in Singapore developed encephalitis. The abattoir had imported pigs from a Malaysian farm. One man died.

'People were falling ill and we had to do something', said Dr Tee Ah Siam, Deputy Director of the Disease Control Division at the Malaysian Health Ministry. The authorities concluded that this was an outbreak of Japanese encephalitis. JE is a mosquito-borne infection that can cause identical symptoms to any other form of encephalitis; it has been around in Malaysia for at least forty-five years. The diagnosis seemed to be confirmed by the fact that many of the victims were involved with pig farming. JE can infect pigs, causing miscarriages among pregnant sows. Pig farmers and their pigs were hurriedly vaccinated against JE, as was anyone living or working within 2km of a pig farm; farms were fumigated to eradicate the mosquitoes. Dr Henry Too, a swine expert from Malaysia's Universiti Putra Faculty of Veterinary Medicine, explained, 'For a disease that causes neurological disorders affecting people who are associated with pigs, JE was a logical presumptive diagnosis' during the early days of the outbreak, based on the fact that it was the only documented disease that affects the brain of those who work with pigs. Furthermore, JE shows seasonal peaks in about November, much as in this episode.

Something, though, was horribly wrong. The measures taken were simply ineffective. Vaccinated pig farmers became ill and died anyway. The vicious spread of the lethal disease continued unchecked. Besides, something else didn't add up. During the outbreaks, pigs in Seremban and Tambun developed breathing difficulties and encephalitis, and subsequently died. This was quite unlike JE. Further, it began to be obvious that encephalitis was killing the wrong people. JE tends to kill children and the elderly, whereas this outbreak was killing young adults, and too many of them. JE normally has a mortality of between 10 per cent and an absolute maximum of 50 per cent; this episode had a mortality in excess of 50 per cent. An emergency regional conference was held in

Ipoh in February 1999 on JE. The Kinta district health officer, Dr Marina, who had originally been convinced that JE was to blame, said that it was 'puzzling' that 80 per cent of patients in Perak were adults. Nor did anyone seem to be able to isolate the JE virus consistently from many of the sick patients. There was absolutely no indisputable proof that the outbreak really was caused by JE. Malaysia is familiar with JE, so this should have been straightforward. Mary Jane Cardosa, head of Universiti Malaysia Sarawak's Institute of Health and Community Medicine, noticed something else that didn't fit. The incidence of the disease in humans paralleled the occurrence of the disease in pigs. If JE were to blame, then mosquitoes would have transmitted it to other victims unconnected with swine. Yet the infected pigs seemed to be the main and, perhaps, only source of infections in humans.

By the time the outbreak had spread to another district, to Negeri Sembilan in early 1999, it became all too obvious that the illness, in pigs at any rate, simply could not be JE. Vets and farm owners began to report that the sows were coughing, panting like dogs, shaking their heads in pain and attacking one another. Shortly after, they would suffer fits and then die, with blood oozing from their snouts. Even farmers familiar with JE began to question the official line. A few days after the Ipoh JE conference, it was announced that the JE virus had been found in only four of twenty-five fatal cases between October and March. By then, expert help had been called in from the Centers for Disease Control in Atlanta, Georgia, led by Dr Thomas Ksiazek. By mid-March, the team had something important to report.

An entirely new virus had been isolated. It was named 'Nipah', after the region in which it was found. Nipah is a paramyxovirus, like measles. It is sufficiently different from any other virus to be given its own genus, *Henipavirus*.

Despite overwhelming evidence that JE was not responsible for the outbreak, the powers that be still could not overcome their convictions. For a time, the virus was still called JE/Nipah. Even as the announcement was made, Health Ministry Director-General Abu Bakar Datuk Suleiman defended the JE diagnosis: 'We are unsure of the role of the Hendra-like virus in the outbreak', he said. No advice to farmers to stop handling their pigs was issued.

Eventually, however, facts had to be faced. Controlling the disease was possible only by a mass cull of infected animals. Slaughtering 1.1 million suspected infected pigs finally halted the march of the disease. The last reported cluster occurred in the south, in Sungai Buloh, in 1999.

Where did the infection come from? If the disease had spread from one species to another, it seemed reasonable to suppose that a third might be involved. A variety of rainforest fauna was tested. Five species of flying foxes, also known as fruit bats, of the genus *Pteropus* were found to have antibodies to Nipah. The presence of antibodies in healthy animals suggested that the bats acquired the infection naturally, yet were immune to it. They shed the live virus in their stools, which then dropped into the pig pens. Nipah caused encephalitis in the pigs, who then bit one another. They also developed respiratory infections and coughed over one another, readily transmitting the contagion. At the time, scientists were relieved that the terrifying possibility that the virus might pass from human to human was not realised.

In Meherpur and Naogaon, Bangladesh between 2001 and 2003, there were twenty-five cases of Nipah. In January and February 2004, forty-seven more became infected in two outbreaks; thirty-five of these died. This represented a 74 per cent mortality rate, despite some patients being given ribavirin, a drug effective against many viruses. Naturally, a link with swine was sought; this was not found. A cluster of five cases in the village of Chandpur, Meherpur occurred in persons from the same household as one of the first to be affected; the cluster consisted of the index patient's wife, son, brother and sister. In Meherpur, pigs and bats were tested for Nipah; none was positive. In Naogaon, two bats tested positive, but no birds, dogs, rodents or pigs. Contact with sick cows was found to be a risk factor, but did not explain the family cluster. This detailed study, by a team which included the American group which had first identified the new virus, drew the shocking conclusion that the disease may be spread between humans. Nipah virus has been detected in respiratory secretions and urine of patients, which suggests that person-to-person transmission is possible.

Nor is Nipah confined to the Malaysian peninsula, nor to pigs and bats. In 1994–5, an unexplained illness killed fifteen horses in Queensland, Australia. Two people also died. In January 1999, another horse died near Cairns. A research team at the Australian Animal Health Laboratory was detailed to isolate and identify the cause. Once again, a measles-like virus of the *Paramyxoviridae* family was isolated. This was initially called equine morbillivirus, and was thought to be similar to the canine distemper virus. This type of illness had never previously been found to kill both horses and humans. When the genetic code of the infection was cracked, it was reclassified in a new genus within the *Paramyxoviridae*. It was renamed Hendra, after the Brisbane suburb in which the first outbreak had occurred. It is almost identical to Nipah.

As with Nipah, Hendra may be found naturally in Australian *Pteropus* fruitbats. Once it transmits to horses and humans, it becomes far more unpleasant. Fever can develop, along with respiratory difficulty and a blood-tinged foamy discharge from the nose and mouth – the virus damages blood vessels. It also induces pulmonary oedema, whereby the lungs fill with fluid. Like the other paramyxoviruses – canine distemper, rinderpest and measles – Hendra virus can cause brain damage. Even more worryingly, cats and guinea pigs may be artificially infected in the laboratory, and can suffer severe disease. Rabbits have also been infected in the laboratory, but do not become ill; this is in a sense more troublesome, as they could therefore become carriers. The very scary conclusion was that domestic pets may become vectors of this horrific new disease. Dogs, chickens, rats and mice do not seem to be susceptible.

Here, then, is a worrying paradigm for humans increasingly encroaching on rainforests. Who knows what other potential threats lie out there, which can leap species and cause untreatable infections in humans? Nipah and Hendra are effectively untreatable. The antiviral ribavirin, which was given to some Nipah victims in the later Malaysian outbreaks, seemed to result in less severe disease, but this was certainly no cure.

As far as we know, these viruses do not seem to mutate between harmless carriage in the fruitbat and lethal infection in horses, pigs and humans. It would seem that they are simply capable of killing susceptible species, and only require an efficient means of transmission through inhalation to wreak their havoc. This is quite unlike bird flu, for example, which at the time of writing actually needs to change its genetic make-up before it can cause a major outbreak.

This leads us neatly to the next of our new Quiet Killers, the human immunodeficiency virus. The origin and indeed definition of HIV as a 'new' disease will now be examined. Way back in the early days of the infection, all manner of wild theories were floated to try to explain this cruel disease. There seemed to be an association with the wilder clubbing scene among gay men – for a time, amyl or butyl nitrate 'poppers' were blamed. These were inhaled to provide an added frisson to orgasm. Others suggested that the disease was deliberate poisoning by some right-wing fundamentalist cadre determined to punish the gay world for their profligate lifestyle.

It rapidly became clear that one of the Quiet Killers was to blame. In June 1982, that conclusion was drawn when a report of a group of cases among gay men in southern California was published. It suggested, for the first time, that the disease was caused by something infectious that was sexually transmitted; the very first reports of clusters of unusual cancers and infections in gay men had appeared in March 1981. By December 1982, reports of transmission by blood transfusion and from mother to foetus had been made, settling the issue for good. These two observations alone almost satisfy the famous Koch's postulates.

But what was this disease? In May 1983, doctors at the Institut Pasteur in France reported that they had found a new virus, which they called lymphadenopathy-associated virus or LAV. The reception of the news was surprisingly downbeat, given that by the end of 1983 the number of AIDS cases in the United States had risen to 3,064 with 1,292 deaths. Nonetheless, specimens were sent to the CDC in Atlanta and to the National Cancer Institute. It wasn't until 22 April 1984 that a spokesman for the CDC was reported as saying: 'I believe we have the cause of AIDS.' He was referring to the French virus. On 23 April, the United States Health and Human Services Secretary Margaret Heckler announced that Dr Robert Gallo of the National Cancer Institute had isolated the virus which caused AIDS. He had called it HTLV-III. By January 1985, it had become clear that LAV and HTLV-III were one and the same.

Identifying the virus did not stop the conspiracy theorists, because at this point there was no convincing evidence to show where it had come from. A significant number of African Americans still believe to this day that HIV was deliberately created by the CIA, in conjunction with the Special Cancer Virus Program, to wipe out large numbers of black and homosexual people. Others blame the smallpox inoculation programme, or claim that gay men were deliberately infected through hepatitis B vaccine trials. The evidence for these theories is negligible. A more convincing hypothesis was contamination of the oral polio vaccine; Edward Hooper, a journalist, wrote a book called *The River*, in which he suggested that HIV could be traced to the testing of an oral polio vaccine called CHAT. This trial vaccine was given to about one million people in Central Africa in the late 1950s. Hooper believed that CHAT was grown in chimpanzee kidney cells infected with a virus similar to HIV called SIV (S for Simian). His intriguing theory ran into the ground when the Wistar Institute was able to find stored specimens of its original vaccine. Not only was it negative for HIV and SIV, but the vaccine was found to have been grown on macaque kidney cells. These cannot be infected with SIV or HIV.

Is the virus really new, and where did it come from? Evidence that the virus has been around for a while, and was circulating naturally among humans in the past, would damage some conspiracy theories well below the waterline. This especially applies to the hypothesis that maintains that HIV is man-made. HIV detection technology has advanced since LAV and HTLV-III were described. The virus can now be sub-typed. It is possible to plot the evolution of sub-types mathematically and thus estimate more or less when the infection first appeared in humans. The current best computer model estimate suggests that the first case of HIV-I infection occurred around 1930, give or take fifteen years, in West Africa. Further evidence comes from stored specimens. A plasma sample taken in 1959 from the Democratic Republic of Congo, and tissue samples from an American teenager who died in St Louis in 1969 and a Norwegian sailor who died around 1976 have all tested positive for HIV. Some scientists who have examined data from the 1959 sample believe infection may date from as early as the late 1800s. Intriguingly, a mutation that protects from HIV infection has been found in Bronze-Age skeletons.

Could the virus have come from outer space, as some said, attached to a meteorite? This is an unlikely explanation. Viruses are often susceptible to ultraviolet light; survival in the extreme heat of penetration of Earth's atmosphere would also make extraterrestrial contamination unlikely. Here is the most current, widely held and scientifically valid explanation.

HIV is variously classified as a lentivirus, or a retrovirus. It is not the only example of its type; there are retroviruses in many animal species, including cats, seals and primates. There are other retroviruses that infect humans, some of which are very unpleasant. Others are harmless, and may even be beneficial (see Chapter Six). Transmission between species has conventionally been thought to be very unusual, if not impossible. However, evidence published in *The Lancet* in 2004 demonstrated that retroviruses may transmit from primates to humans, and that such transfer is still happening. Scientists in that study looked at 1,099 people from Cameroon. They found that ten of them had blood evidence of simian foamy virus. This retrovirus had not previously been thought to infect humans. The theory is that the mingling of blood which might occur during the brutal butchering of bush meat might permit such an inoculation. Some monkeys carry a retrovirus called SIVcpz. It is now thought that this virus was transferred to hunting humans by the same route. Many think that bushmeat should be banned for this reason.

Various compounding factors peculiar to Africa have been suggested as facilitating the initial transfer of this new infection into humans. Widespread sharing of needles in impoverished African clinics and hospitals would have not only ensured effective transmission, but also permitted 'passage' of viruses through living subjects. Each time the virus infected a new host, it would react differently with each individual's immune system. A totally new virus would result; the eventual consequence could feasibly be a virus specially adapted for survival in humans. Others suggest that colonialism has contributed, particularly the peculiarly brutal variety practised by the French and Belgians in Central Africa. In the early years of the twentieth century, camps of forced labour were established, where the natives were malnourished and overworked. It has emerged that some of these camps had 50 per cent mortality; records were subsequently systematically erased. Bushmeat would have been welcome to these unfortunate victims of inhumanity; it is possible that debilitated and poorly fed slave labourers might have been more susceptible to viral infection, and that interaction with the immune system of someone already ill might have different outcomes for both human and virus. This would tally with our mathematical prediction for the origin of the first HIV strains.

It would also contain a prophetic echo for the subsequent course of the pandemic. There is little doubt that poverty and injustice continue to compound the effects of this terrible scourge. Treatments for HIV are widely available in the West; in the developing world, they have been only procurable for the privileged few. AIDS – the constellation of infections and cancers which develop as a result of unchecked HIV infection – is thus a preventable condition in developed nations. In a sense, it is therefore poverty which causes AIDS in some parts of the world, not HIV. Making the drugs generally and cheaply available may have its own unfortunate consequences, as we have discussed.

The notion of HIV as a 'new' disease is, therefore, open to interpretation. Its novelty is almost exactly balanced between two clichés: there is nothing new under the sun; and always something new out of Africa. The same principle, though, emerges: when humans encroach on new habitats, we risk exposing ourselves to different Quiet Killers.

In such a case the disease is only recognised when sufficiently large populations are exposed to generate a cluster. Once the cause is

identified, it becomes apparent that the disease is not new after all –
animal reservoirs are found; once the disease is sought more
assiduously, it becomes obvious that there are many other cases;
review of the historical records shows that it has been encountered
before, but the technology was not available to characterise it. This
was precisely the sequence in the emergence of Lyme disease, a
condition spread by ticks which causes arthritis and rash, often
among children. It kills so rarely that it hardly belongs among the
Quiet Killers, but it is worth noting that the diagnosis of this new
disease arose when there was an unexpected cluster of arthritis
among children in a small geographical area – Old Lyme,
Connecticut in the United States.

There is another 'new' Quiet Killer which does not obey these
rules, and it is in many ways a scary one. Its symptoms arrive
insidiously. There are many throughout the world who are unaware
that they are infected and so run the risk of passing the infection on
to their loved ones; worryingly, its routes of spread are unclear – no
one is certain how some people caught it. Many doctors think of
this infection as a time bomb because it may lie dormant for so long
and there is such a huge reservoir of silent, infectious cases. When it
awakes, it can cause liver failure, cancer and a myriad of other
symptoms including chronic fatigue and arthritis. As far as we
know, there is no animal reservoir or vector. As a disease, it emerged
only about fifteen years ago, and it was identified only because there
was a gap in the alphabet. For many years the list was effectively
hepatitis A, hepatitis B, hepatitis D and then non-A, non-B. We now
know this as hepatitis C.

In clinics, it was often hard to spot what had happened in the lives
of patients with hepatitis C to allow this Quiet Killer to intrude. We
know that blood transfusion used to be a source (until screening was
introduced) and many haemophiliacs were early sufferers, picking up
the infection through contaminated, pooled blood products. People
who had injected recreational drugs into themselves were also at
risk. But there was a definite cohort of middle-aged men and women
whose lives appeared relatively innocuous. A common – but not
exclusive – factor appeared to be youth during the latter 1960s. As is

sometimes said, if you can remember the sixties, you probably weren't there. It is possible that the relaxation of sexual mores during those heady decades allowed readier transmission of a virus that can pass by the venereal route. The illness seemed to me a heavy price to pay for a few years of carnal experimentation. Indeed, some even dispute the sexual route as a means of transmission, although the evidence seems in favour. Certain vigorous sexual practices have been shown to favour the transmission of the disease, but I found it hard to match practices such as these with some of the personalities I was treating. Transmission between monogamous heterosexual couples is very rare, although it does happen. The virus just isn't very good at getting from person to person. Even pregnant infected mothers transmit the disease to their babies rarely, in only about 10 per cent of cases.

All this makes the figures for numbers affected all the more startling. Approximately 170 million people worldwide and 4 million in the United States are infected with hepatitis C. Given that there is no known animal source of the disease, and that it is not an easy virus to catch, these figures are astonishing. Due to the silent nature of infection – this really is a Quiet Killer – there are many who have no idea that they are infected. The figures amount to tens of thousands in Britain alone. Some of these will only discover that they are infected when they develop liver failure or liver cancer in later life. The risks are increased by drinking alcohol. A proportion will die before any symptoms develop, but in about a third cirrhosis will arise during life.

Hepatitis C is related to Yellow Fever and West Nile viruses, being a flavivirus. Hepatitis C was discovered in 1989 by investigators at a drug company called Chiron, Inc. They made their discovery following the observation that patients who had received blood transfusions were still developing prolonged hepatitis that was neither A nor B, and despite careful screening. The method they used was clever and elegant: they infected a chimpanzee with serum from an infected patient, then observed all the DNA products from the chimp's genes. They observed some extra fragments that other chimps did not share, and reasoned that these must be the virus. To this day, it is not feasible to culture the virus in the lab, a fact which has hampered development of treatments.

The origins of the hepatitis C epidemic remain something of a mystery. Making use of the so-called 'molecular clock', a calculation based on the rate of mutation of the genes within the RNA, allows for some speculation. The current leading hypothesis suggests that it arose in widespread form about sixty to seventy years ago, quite abruptly. A vaguely similar virus has been identified in a tamarind monkey, but is not close enough to imply transmission to humans. However, hepatitis C is one of the most genetically diverse viruses identified to date, implying that it has been around for far longer. This in turn implies a very important question: if the virus is largely spread by blood contact, how did it persist among humans before transfusion and injecting drug use were commonplace? Tribal tattooing rites and insect vectors have been suggested, but there is no proof. This genetic diversity is of more than academic interest – some genotypes are far less susceptible to current treatments than others. The best treatment available at present is a combination of the naturally occurring antiviral chemical interferon with the drug ribavirin, over prolonged periods. The treatment often causes side effects and has a cure rate only in the order of 50 to 80 per cent, depending on the infecting strain.

* * *

Some 'new' infections may lie far closer than you think. There is a fair chance – up to 10 per cent – that your plumbing may harbour a threat that was unknown until 1976, and since then has killed hundreds worldwide. Even if you do not have air conditioning, this lethal bacterium may lurk in your shower head or central heating; or in the hot tub or swimming pool of your local gymnasium. Many will be familiar with *Legionella pneumophila* from the famous outbreak at the American military legionnaires' convention in Philadelphia. You are less likely to be familiar with the peculiar and complex life cycle of this fastidious bacterium, or with the diligence and ingenuity of the team that solved the puzzle of that outbreak.

You may think that a disease described in 1976 barely counts as 'new' any more. In evolutionary terms, and on the schedule of the Quiet Killers, to whom time is an irrelevance, 1976 is still today. Legionnaires' disease also illustrates a number of key issues about new infections, such as where they come from; whether we have met them before; whether they are truly new; and how even simple changes in our behaviour can expose us to new threats. The extraordinary story of the discovery of *Legionella pneumophila* reads in many ways more like something from Agatha Christie than *The Lancet*.

The 1976 Convention of the American Legion was intended to be memorable and historic for one reason alone. It was the bicentennial meeting of the association, marking 200 years since the War of Independence. It was the Legion's 58th convention. The three-day event was billed to commence on 21 July 1976 at the Bellevue Stratford Hotel, Philadelphia, and involved more than 4,000 ex-Second World War servicemen and their families. About 600 of the former servicemen stayed at the Bellevue. Many would not live to regret this decision.

From the outset, there was a spectre at the feast. The convention was meant to be a celebration of fellowship and survival through adversity. However, almost immediately after the inaugural ceremony, illness began to strike. One by one, delegates began to complain of fever, pains in the chest, cough and breathlessness. The first death occurred four days after the convention ended, on Tuesday 27 July. At the final tally, 221 people had been infected, and 34 had died.

Responsibility for the investigation of this kind of outbreak lies with the Centers for Disease Control (CDC) in Atlanta, Georgia. This organisation was already on edge in 1976. The CDC was expecting a flu outbreak; they initially drew the conclusion that the Philadelphia disease was just that. The organisation was war-weary itself following a prolonged battle in Congress over vaccination for a possible influenza epidemic earlier that year; the death of a soldier from Influenza A at Fort Dix looked like a straw in the wind for a gathering storm. But none of the tests for influenza from the developing problem in Philadelphia was positive. Something else was going on;

the only thing that the scientists could agree on, ironically as it turned out, was that this was not a bacterial disease. Nonetheless, mass influenza vaccination was commenced in October 1976.

Without a conclusive diagnosis, conspiracy theories inevitably began to pop up. All that the CDC were really able to say was that there seemed to be some sort of association with the hotel lobby, where many of the victims had congregated or loitered to smoke cigarettes. The conspiracy theorists scoffed at this apparently meaningless association. Some believed that the legionnaires were being assassinated by communists or drug companies. Various poisons, including nickel, were suggested. Matters became worse when complications of the mass flu vaccination programme developed. Several elderly people died, and others developed neurological diseases related to the vaccine. Eventually, the programme was abandoned.

The CDC understandably cast their net wide in their search for a cause. Specimens were sent to the laboratory of Dr Joseph McDade. His particular interest was a group of organisms called the *Rickettsiae*. We have met them before, as ancestors of our mitochondria and vital parts of ourselves. They are tiny, incomplete bacteria that cause a range of illnesses from typhus to Q-fever, an unpleasant and chronic illness of man and sheep. Q-fever can be hard to diagnose. Q actually stands for Query, because the nature of the disease was for so long obscure. Such diseases are best investigated by the meticulous and the near obsessive, such as McDade.

McDade found that the tissues from victims caused fever and a fatal illness when inoculated into guinea pigs. One of Koch's postulates confirming the cause of a disease – passage through animals – was thus confirmed. The trouble was, he couldn't find that cause. He spotted a few rather sickly looking bacteria in the guinea pig tissues under the microscope; such observations are not uncommon. It is sometimes difficult to discriminate between real disease-causing bacteria and tiny clumps of tissue, artificial stain and contaminants. However, when he tried to encourage the bacteria to grow even in the super-rich medium of embryonated hens' eggs, they simply refused.

McDade is a fastidious, driven and thorough man; his frustration at being so close to the cause of the mysterious disease drew him back to the lab on the evening of 28 December 1976, while all of his colleagues were partying away the end of the year. He decided to take out his guinea pig slides to double-check them. This time he spotted something different. Not artefacts, not stain clumps. Definite bacteria. And inside a white blood cell, exactly where you would expect to see *Rickettsiae*. McDade decided to inoculate these tiny bacilli into the hens' eggs again; this time, he decided to give them their best chance of survival by omitting the antibiotics that supplemented the hens' eggs to suppress contaminating bacteria. Extracts of these eggs were then reintroduced to the guinea pigs. They became ill and died. From then, it was a simple matter to culture and characterise the bacterium. It was named *Legionella* in honour of its early victims. McDade had cracked it.

The question now was, how did these bacteria get into people, and why was this particular hotel so clearly implicated? What was it about the lobby that was so dangerous? A microbiologist called Dr Carl Fliermans took up the next part of the trail. He realised that *L. pneumophila* in many respects resembled heat-loving bacteria that he'd found in the volcanic geothermal regions of the Yellowstone National Park. These so-called thermophilic bacteria lived in aquatic environments in symbiosis with algae. Dr Fliermans began to look elsewhere, and soon found similar organisms in the cooling water effluent from the nuclear Savannah River Laboratory. Before long, he had identified *Legionella* and similar bacteria in just about every aquatic environment in the United States, as well as in virtually every cooling tower and, of course, air conditioning systems. Basically, where there is warm mist, there are algae and there are thermophilic bacteria, including *Legionella*. The air conditioning unit is an almost exact reproduction of an ancient ecological niche.

Legionella pneumophila is, in some respects, halfway between a virus and a bacterium. Like a virus, it cannot easily survive on its own. Unlike other bacteria – *Pseudomonas* for example, which will grow almost anywhere – it is extremely choosy about where it will set up shop. It needs the life-support system of more complex organisms to exist. This is true of its state in nature, in the laboratory and in infection. In the body, the germ allows itself to be enveloped by white blood cells. It has mechanisms to prevent attack by the deadly bleach-like substance that white blood cells use to annihilate invaders. It can then live and reproduce in the nutrient-rich environment inside the cell. In the lab, it will not grow on ordinary agar. This is how picky it is: it needs to be supplemented with precise extracts of yeast buffered to an exact acidity; at higher than usual temperatures; and with high levels of the amino acid cysteine, plus inorganic iron supplements, low sodium concentrations, and activated charcoal to absorb free radicals. It may grow when inoculated into an animal – and even then, only certain animals will do. In the wild, it lives inside some bizarre and complex life forms, some of which are only just being discovered, and in specific conditions of humidity and temperature.

These life forms are crucial to the way in which we have now begun to encounter *Legionella* as a Quiet Killer, because it is their habitat which we have disturbed. *Tetrahymena pyriformis* is a protozoon. It likes two things: a warm, moist environment and eating bacteria. One of the bacteria it likes to eat is *Legionella pneumophila*. Its lifestyle requirements mean that it loves exactly the kind of lukewarm moist environment found in stagnant water in hot tubs and swimming pools. Its eating habits mean that it provides a comfortable home for one of our Quiet Killers. The combination provides a vehicle that can only really afflict modern humans. Central heating systems, swimming pools, air conditioning units, hot tubs with water recirculated through pumps that can cause aerosols – these are all modern, twentieth-century inventions.

Two major conclusions about legionellosis could be drawn from the information that it occurs in nature and that it was transmitted, in the Philadelphia outbreak, via air conditioning units. The first is that not all of the victims of the 1976 outbreak would have been legionnaires; anyone passing by the air conditioning vent might have been infected. Sure enough, when the data were re-analysed, 72 of the 221 victims had simply either walked past the hotel lobby or had stayed coincidentally at the Bellevue Stratford. The second conclusion was that other, previously unexplained respiratory illnesses might have been due to *Legionella*. It seemed reasonable to look at the same site – and sure enough, two years before, in 1974, eleven members of an Oddfellows convention staying at the Bellevue Stratford Hotel had become ill; tests revealed *Legionella* to be the cause. There are two forms of infection with the bacterium: the pneumonia and a flu-like illness with a far lower mortality, known as Pontiac Fever; a further illness undiagnosed in 1968 was subsequently identified in Pontiac, Michigan, and gave this variant its name. Doctors also recalled an unexplained illness in a psychiatric hospital in Washington DC in 1965, in which there were 15 deaths. Blood specimens were stored from that episode. Almost all (85 per cent) tested positive for legionnaires' disease.

In a curious aside, an entirely new life form was discovered as a consequence of research into *Legionella*. A British scientist called Tim Rowbotham was studying the microbiology of cooling towers in 1992. He was interested in which *Legionella* infected which protozoa. He found *Legionella* particles in amoebae isolated from a Bradford industrial cooling tower. The genetic make-up of these amoebae appeared quite unique. He named his new organism *Bradfordcoccus*. This was a totally new type of animal. The cooling tower has subsequently been knocked down and science may have lost the only colony of his odd life form. As this story illustrates, we are far indeed from identifying the nature and life cycles of even such organisms which are on our doorstep, let alone within the oceans or wildernesses of the world. Many of the bacteria in our own mouths still defy identification. We almost certainly have not identified the last of our Quiet Killers.

This chapter has focused on those particular 'new' diseases that illustrate the general nature of novel infections, why they arise and how they were identified. Of course, it is not an exhaustive list, and what seems new today will be old hat tomorrow. What are the diseases, though, that we can expect to encounter in the future? The final chapter of this book will seek to answer this question.

ELEVEN

The Future

To my current knowledge, there is no cohort of unwell patients lurking, awaiting a diagnosis of a previously unencountered Quiet Killer. However, that is not to say there are no new infectious agents to be identified.

It is impossible to predict which new infectious diseases will trouble us in the coming years. However, there are certain principles that are indicative of where and how such diseases would arise:

1. A 'new' infection is far more likely to be a virus than a bacterium, a worm or a fungus. I have several reasons for saying this. First, history. Almost all of the recent 'new' diseases have been viruses – Nipah, Hendra, West Nile, avian flu, HIV. The exception is new variant CJD, which belongs to none of the categories, being neither bacterium nor virus nor any previously recognisable agent. Second, viruses have a far higher rate of mutation, which makes novel varieties of infection more common. Third, because the techniques for detecting viruses have until recently been much more difficult than those to detect bacteria, the chances of a virus being 'missed' are higher. Lastly, in general viruses transmit far more readily than bacteria or the other agents from person to person, or from animals to humans.

2. The infection will come from animals, but will be capable of spreading between people. Almost all of the new infections listed above have arisen from contact with animals, and the optimal agent for widespread transmission of disease from animals to humans is a virus. Although transmission of bacteria, fungi and worms from animals to humans is common,

the chain is usually short. TB may be the exception to this rule, being a bacterial infection that may have arisen initially in cattle. However, new epidemic varieties of TB are unlikely, as unlike viruses the bacterium evolves very slowly. Viruses form small particles, by their very nature, which disseminate easily.

3. The new infection will arise in a developing country where the public health surveillance system is rudimentary and where economics demand that natural resources must be exploited to the full. This is related to my second point. It is within the developing countries that rainforests are being invaded and exploited as never before, and the gross changes in local ecology can cause diseases to change their behaviour.

Beyond these broad predictions, it is hard to make any definitive statement about new diseases. One could speculate that flaviviruses would be likely candidates, having been responsible for hepatitis C and West Nile Fever, as well as Yellow Fever, which, although it is not 'new', perfectly illustrates point 3 above. It is also possible that we may fall victim to an 'Andromeda Strain' – an infection from outer space, as outlined in Michael Crichton's novel of the same name. However, I think this unlikely. Apart from the technical difficulties involved with living material surviving re-entry on mineral tissue like meteorites, it has been a feature of the Quiet Killers that we have discussed that they co-evolved either with humans or with animals on our planet. For a suitable infectious agent to transmit from space, we would have to postulate a living host sufficiently similar to animal life on another planet for such evolution to occur. Of course this is entirely possible – in theory.

There are other possibilities for the discovery of new infections. We could call this the 'New Applications for Old Diseases' theory. This is the discovery of infection as the cause of illness where none was previously expected or proven. An example of this is the discovery of the bacterium that is now widely believed to be the cause of stomach ulcers and some varieties of stomach cancer, *Helicobacter pylori*. The announcement that this was the possible cause of the condition was met with disbelief to the point of derision in some quarters; now, it is almost universally accepted.

Nonetheless, it is my conjecture that many illnesses will be shown to have at least partly an infectious cause. The list is already impressive. This phenomenon has been demonstrated in the following cancers, with the causative agents in brackets: cervical cancer (human papilloma virus); Kaposi's sarcoma (human herpes virus 8); mucosal-associated lymphoid tumours (*Helicobacter pylori*); Castleman's disease (human herpes virus 6); nasopharyngeal carcinoma and Burkitt's lymphoma (Epstein-Barr virus); adult T-cell lymphoma/leukaemia (human T-cell lymphotrophic virus I).

Many doctors believe that it is only a matter of time before the infectious agent behind the unpleasant neurological condition multiple sclerosis is identified. There are a number of pieces of circumstantial evidence to support this view. Sufferers may be shown to have had higher than average numbers of respiratory infections compared to non-sufferers; the disease occurs in clusters in susceptible communities, exactly like other infections; there was a famous 'epidemic'-like appearance and disappearance of a cluster of cases on the Faroe Islands. Just about every antibiotic and antiviral agent has been tested for multiple sclerosis; numerous agents have been suggested as causes from rabies to Marek's Semliki forest virus. To date, no serious candidate has come forward. The notion of an infectious cause has been around for a very long time. The French scientist Pierre Marie postulated such a process as long ago as 1894. He could not cite a specific organism as cause, but predicted the eventual development of a vaccine. Sadly, his prediction has been way off the mark so far.

Chlamydia – a group of bacteria that cause a range of illnesses from sexually transmitted infections to pneumonia to blindness and possibly heart attacks – has been top of the shortlist for some years, as has Epstein-Barr virus, the agent of glandular fever. While there may be some circumstantial evidence to support both, the real proof has eluded us. It may be that the associations are a statistical quirk, or even that the disease process that makes victims susceptible to MS also means that they are more vulnerable to infections with these agents.

Nevertheless, just because an infectious agent has not been identified does not mean that there isn't one. Absence of proof is not the same as proof of absence. There are a number of diseases whose effects arise even after the Quiet Killer has gone on its way. Rheumatic fever is just such an example; another is a rare brain disorder following infection with the common bacterium *Mycoplasma pneumoniae*. This agent commonly causes pneumonia; subsequently, some patients develop an unpleasant encephalitis which does not respond to the antibiotic active against the original agent, because it has gone. Ekiri syndrome is a very similar disease which arises after dysentery with *Shigella sonnei*. Reiter's syndrome, a mixture of arthritis and eye inflammation, may occur after sexually transmitted diseases. An extremely unpleasant paralysis called Guillain-Barré syndrome may develop after infection with the common diarrhoea bacterium *Campylobacter* (among others). I have mentioned the potential disastrous long-term consequences of measles infection. The point of this list is that the consequences of a visit from a Quiet Killer may be delayed; this may explain why multiple sclerosis may not respond to antiviral (or antibacterial) drugs even if they are directed at the correct cause. The illness itself may be autoimmune; the infectious trigger causes the body to attack itself and the damage persists and continues after the trigger has gone. It is worth noting, though, that Stanley Prusiner, who won the Nobel Prize for his work on prions in BSE, does not include MS in his list of diseases that he considers to be caused by an infection.

There are other diseases which are strongly suspected or known to have an infectious component. Heart disease and diabetes may have one. Some have speculated that even obesity may be made more likely by viral triggers. Many more are likely to come forward.

The most frightening challenge for the twenty-first century inevitably involves bioterrorism. The possibility that advanced laboratories may modify a deadly infection like smallpox to make it resistant to vaccines is a terrifying theoretical possibility. Exactly the same technology that has been used to develop better understanding of bacteria, fungi and viruses, and to harness them to produce useful products may be employed to make dangerous organisms even more lethal. Yeasts may easily be genetically modified to produce insulin for diabetics or Factor VIII for haemophiliacs in industrial quantities and to very stringent standards of purity. The method of doing so is to identify the correct gene from a human or animal source, and then to splice that segment into a rapidly reproducing yeast. Imagine what could be done to evil ends with the same technology. We are daily immersed in harmless organisms. Suppose someone were to splice a gene which encodes a deadly property into an otherwise harmless common virus? Suppose someone were to take a virus like smallpox and alter its genetic structure such that the vaccine no longer worked? The series of blunders, coincidences, unethical experiments and near-disasters that led to the development of a smallpox vaccine has already been discussed. There is simply no way that this could be repeated in the modern world, although one has to allow that desperation in the face of an unstoppable epidemic might make a virtue out of the unthinkable. The ability to splice and re-assort genes means that a skilled scientist could simply select the qualities of their weapon like picking items from a supermarket shelf, even creating a totally new virus which mankind had never encountered before.

*   *   *

Humankind will undoubtedly face greater challenges in the future from infectious diseases: more resistance to antibiotics; new diseases; old diseases in new places. We know about some of the mistakes we made in the twentieth century that allowed a Golden Age of protection from infection to slip through our fingers. Can we claw any of it back? Is there anything new on the horizon that might tip the balance in our favour again?

The continuing struggle between humans and the Quiet Killers is like an ungloved boxing match between two prize-fighters; looked at over history, both have exchanged near-killer blows but neither has quite had the other out for the count. Nor will either ever. At the moment, it looks like it is we who are on the back foot. Drug-resistant HIV disease, TB, MRSA, malaria – each is a real hazard;

the further dangers of new emerging diseases such as Nipah and Influenza A in the form of epidemics transmitted through animals such as birds are ever with us.

Humans will always be stalked by the Quiet Killers. Yet humankind is not a hapless, feckless or passive victim in this prize fight. First, it has to be remembered that the Quiet Killers are nowhere near re-establishing themselves as the scourges they once were. In Chapter One, we discussed their former pre-eminence as a cause of death. In population terms, the emergence of resistance has led to individual, small-scale tragedy rather than mass slaughter. The simple fact is that most infections remain curable in a healthy victim. This makes the continuing death toll from treatable infections in the developing world ever more shameful.

Next, we must recall that we have met the new challenges with effective and timely weapons. Hepatitis C was only identified in 1985. Already we have treatments which provide a cure in a significant proportion of victims. That number steadily increases as existing technology is used more efficiently. Initially, the rate of cure was in the order of 40 per cent; the best results from using combination treatments of newer interferon preparations combined with the antiviral drug ribavirin now means that more than 60 per cent may be cured. Even those in whom treatment has failed are now being offered treatments unthinkable a generation ago; liver transplantation for hepatitis C is almost routine in some countries. Less radical alternatives to the major surgery involved – injecting preparations of immature liver cells – are being successfully pioneered. New agents are being developed as I write; this will be discussed in more detail below. The Nipah virus outbreak in South-East Asia was controlled once the cause was correctly identified, not by a miracle 'silver bullet' drug, but by old-fashioned principles of public health control that would have been clearly understood in the century before last. Many nations have sophisticated and advanced plans to deal with a possible global pandemic of influenza. These are based on a combination of vaccination, public health containment and anti-flu drugs such as oseltamivir. Such measures might well have prevented the Great Pandemic of 1917–18.

We have real evidence of the creativity of man when faced with a new challenge. The pace of change in treatments for the 'new' epidemic of HIV/AIDS has been breathtaking. From the beginning of the pandemic until 1996, all too often doctors could only observe the inexorable decline and death of victims. Although they could treat many of the infections that ravaged decimated immune systems, the eventual outcome seemed inevitable. In one ward where I worked, there was a book of condolence that relatives, staff and friends would use to record their memories as tragedy followed tragedy. In those days, the book needed replacing on a frequent basis; deaths were almost a daily occurrence. By the late 1990s, however, the situation had changed completely; the book of condolence hardly ever needed replacing. The ward was almost empty; in fact, one half had to be closed because the number of desperately sick people had fallen so dramatically. What had changed was the introduction of combination treatments for the virus. The penny had dropped – some say, rather belatedly – that the virus mutated so rapidly that single drugs became ineffective almost immediately. What was needed was a combination, usually of at least three. Suppressing the virus allowed the crippled white cells to recover. Practically moribund patients had their health turned around almost overnight. While this method has not been perfect, or even a cure, it is a testament to the ingenuity of humans that a disease discovered only decades before was now no longer an inevitable death sentence. It seems reasonable, if not guaranteed, that we might meet the next Quiet Killer with the same resourcefulness.

There are many caveats, though. The emergence of treatments for HIV was not straightforward, and there were always political pressures involved. Attendees at conferences for HIV and AIDS will recall the demonstrations and protests by sufferers who felt that the world was ignoring their plight; some of these were highly strident. There is also the slightly vexed question of whether such progress could be repeated, and whether it would have been so rapid had the outbreak been confined to the developing world. It has to be acknowledged that even today most research into drugs targeted at HIV is confined to HIV-I, which is the variety that principally infects westerners. HIV-II, the West African variant, is the lesser cousin in research terms; some groups of drugs do not even work against it. Furthermore, many drug companies are scaling down their research programmes generally and anti-infective research specifically. New drug development is a ripe area for litigation; the costs for developing any new medication run into billions of dollars. The delays with large-scale trials and licensing mean that any profits may not be seen for decades. Many drug companies are simply not interested in drugs which are directed at diseases that only affect poor countries or small numbers, nor in producing drugs with low – or unquantifiable – profit potential.

Of course, not all drug companies are calculating or callous, as some medicines are given away free to those who need them. There is an excellent example of this in a drug that is used for a condition which is responsible for one of the commonest causes of blindness in the developing world – onchocerciasis, or river blindness. Examination of the story of this compound, Ivermectin, is extremely instructional in the context of drugs which may give hope for the future. Onchocerciasis is caused by a blood-borne parasite transmitted through the bite of a blackfly. In the 1970s, the most effective method of control, insecticides to kill the blackflies, was beginning to fail. Scientists were looking to improved treatments for people who already had the condition.

The most fruitful source of new anti-infective compounds at that time was the natural world. As we have previously discussed, many organisms produce chemicals to defend themselves. The technique was then to scour suitable environments where bugs were likely to mix with one another and would therefore need to kill their rivals. Fungi were particularly carefully examined, following Fleming's edifying example of penicillin. Soil and sewage outfalls seemed to be the most rich hunting grounds. Oddly though, it was on a golf course in Japan that the anti-parasitic chemical avermectin was discovered. Avermectin was produced by a fungus, *Streptomyces avermitilis*. It was passed on, together with fifty-three other likely compounds, to Merck by the Japanese Kitasato Corporation. Simple modification of the structure of the molecule made it even more effective against parasites. It looked like the company was onto a winner – a safe and effective treatment for a common and debilitating condition; the pharmaceutical Holy Grail.

However, Merck now had something of a problem. Nobody in America, or anywhere in the West, gets river blindness. The countries where people do contract it are poor, and cannot afford expensive drugs. You and I might not think that matters, but companies like Merck have a duty to their shareholders. They cannot pursue commercially non-viable medications on a whim. This is a contentious area, but there are a number of issues to consider here. First, the issuing of medication is not without risk. Supposing Ivermectin had, when prescribed to enough people, caused serious illness in some of them? It may indeed cause complications in another parasitic infection called loaisis. Who would have picked up the legal and compensation bills? Second, supposing there is a superior, safer anti-parasitic agent out there somewhere waiting to be discovered? What would the impetus be for another company to go looking for it if the already feeble market had been saturated by cheap Ivermectin? If Ivermectin were given away free, would other drug companies be expected to do the same with their anti-parasitics? Finally, the alternative to the capitalist approach – state control of drug companies – has signally failed in terms of innovation. No useful new drug was ever invented or developed behind the old Iron Curtain. This is simply a pragmatic truth, although there is a major exception discussed in detail below.

There are, of course, international aid agencies who might reasonably have stepped in at that moment to make Ivermectin widely available. The World Health Organization (WHO), the US Agency for International Development (USAID), and the US Department of State were all approached. It was generally agreed that the effort to cure river blindness was worthwhile, but there was simply no money available to fund a scheme which would have meant complicated delivery of the drug to remote and impoverished countries with poor internal communications. Some US Senators, including Edward Kennedy, wanted congressional action to sponsor free worldwide distribution. The sums could not be found. In 1987,

Merck chairman Dr Roy Vagelos therefore decided that Merck would donate Ivermectin to the world, free of charge, in perpetuity.

By fifteen years after Ivermectin had been made freely available, more than 30 million people were being treated with it each year. Areas that had been rendered uninhabitable by river blindness were once again opened up to human life. The drug is now also used successfully to treat the horribly disfiguring elephantiasis. Treatment of parasitic infections can have unexpected and beneficial consequences; early use of drugs which kill parasites in the intestine has been shown in some studies to improve eventual IQ and height by significant figures.

Would anyone bother to develop Ivermectin for human use today? That is highly debatable. One wonders whether Merck would have pursued the issue had they predicted the final profit-free outcome. Furthermore, our attitude to testing drugs has clearly changed. It is interesting that the original guinea pigs for human Ivermectin use were in Senegal. The morality of western companies' testing of medicines in the developing world has come under intense scrutiny since the AIDS epidemic. All of this is clearly a shame, as Ivermectin is a highly effective and safe drug.

The Ivermectin story does illustrate many of the complexities involved with the hunt for new agents to tackle the Quiet Killers. Drug companies need to have an incentive to pursue research into likely compounds. That incentive is generally financial. Discovery has traditionally been almost serendipitous, like stumbling upon a useful agent on a golf course. While newer technologies have meant that we can attack new targets – we will discuss this later – it is possible that the stock of chance discoveries may be limited.

However, new anti-infective drugs are being invented, and some for use on the most challenging infections. Much has been made of the threat from MRSA. There are several drugs already available or in development for this infection. The newish agent Linezolid remains active against most of the world's MRSA; its problems are that it is more toxic than originally thought and it is expensive. Vancomycin has been the mainstay of MRSA treatment for some years; resistance has emerged, but new derivatives, such as

Oritavancin and Dalbavancin, show great promise. Daptomycin is an antibiotic with an entirely new means of killing bacteria which seems, at the time of writing, to be remarkably safe. Arbekacin has been used with some promise in Japan against both MRSA and VRE, the dangerous hospital pathogen *Enterococcus* which is resistant to Vancomycin. As far as MRSA and VRE are concerned, we are far from being in the last chance saloon.

Nor are new discoveries confined to treatments for bacteria. Whole new classes of antiviral drugs are in development for the AIDS virus, although for each success there is at least one that stumbles. For hepatitis C – partly as a result of the massive increase in knowledge derived from HIV research – a number of new agents, such as the helicases, are under active trial. Vaccines for malaria have shown some promise, and treatment of even highly resistant malaria has been made feasible by the Chinese wormwood derivative artemisinin and chemicals derived from it.

Worryingly, the same may not be true of some of the other bacteria that are prone to multiple resistance. They include *Klebsiella*, *Burkholderia pseudomonas* and EMRAB (Epidemic Multi-Resistant *Acinetobacter baumanii*). These are 'opportunistic' bacteria that generally cause disease in hospitals, among the already sick. They are the scourge of many modern intensive care units and may cause fatal pneumonias, cystitis and wound infections; EMRAB is a particularly problematic bacterium which has led to the temporary closure of more than one intensive care department. Some of these are now genuinely resistant to every known class of conventional antibiotic; they are effectively untreatable. There is one agent, tigecycline, which has been derived by jigging about with the very commonplace antibiotic tetracycline. It is showing promise against some of these opportunistic bacteria, but not really against *pseudomonas*. This is a very important exception. *Pseudomonas* species are extremely versatile and can grow in almost any environment; they even seem to thrive in sterile water. They are a major problem in hospitals, much like our other opportunistic bacteria, and may transfer from medical equipment and the hands of staff into the lungs of patients being artificially ventilated, with fatal results.

It is important to put 'untreatable' bacterial infections into perspective. Only a small number of people suffer with them. That numbers issue is part of the problem, and is of no comfort if you have cystic fibrosis and become infected with *Burkholderia*, or pneumonia from a multi-resistant *pseudomonas*. We need new agents, and we need them soon. The problem is that these conditions are rare and therefore provide little incentive for profit-motivated drug companies to devote expensive research effort into them, especially as regulation of licensing of new drugs becomes increasingly stringent.

So, it is all the fault of so-called Big Pharma – the large pharmaceutical companies – that research into anti-infectives has come off the boil. Isn't it? Many people do hold the drug companies responsible, which is a little unfair. You might consider two major points: large pharmaceutical companies have provided every anti-infective agent now in use; and not every company has abandoned the hunt. For example, both Johnson & Johnson and AstraZeneca are actively seeking new antibiotics, and are also developing novel agents against TB. Some smaller companies have taken up the baton. Daptomycin, for instance, was originally developed by the Big Pharma company Eli Lilly, who shelved it because they didn't think it was effective enough; however, a new company called Cubist is taking it forward. Rather than knocking the pharmaceutical companies, who simply reflect the capitalist environment in which they have thrived, there is a more telling accusation. This charge is levelled at the way in which the major universities are funded; or rather, underfunded. Ask almost any academic and they will ruefully agree that there just isn't enough money around to conduct proper research. There are unfilled professorial chairs in microbiology in Britain for this reason. It might be rewarding to one's self-esteem to become a professor one day, but being a chair with no research money is like being a eunuch in charge of a harem; and one which hasn't even got any women in it. So if academic research is lacking, where will the next generation of anti-infectives come from?

*   *   *

The bald statement that no useful new anti-infective medication ever originated behind the old Iron Curtain needs some qualification. This story is a fascinating one, involving mutual incomprehension between East and West; ideological schism; and scientific and temporal dislocation. Development of phage treatment has teetered between capitalism and communism since their discovery, to the world's loss. Research into phage has been the proving-ground for some of mankind's greatest scientists, and they have hinted at the great key to life. They still yet may offer a degree of hope for the future. And yet, they may be unwittingly dangerous.

We are speaking of bacteriophages. What are they? It has been one of the consistent themes of this book that organisms do not evolve in isolation. As the great satirist Jonathan Swift observed:

> So nat'ralists observe, a flea
> Hath smaller fleas that on him prey;
> And these have smaller still to bite 'em;
> And so proceed *ad infinitum*.

So it is with some of the Quiet Killers. Bacteria feed on other bacteria. Bacteria live inside protozoa, as with our legionnaires' example in the previous chapter. Some bacteria – the genus *Bdellovibrio* – parasitise other bacteria. Some viruses attack and kill bacteria. The latter group comprise the bacteriophages, and it is these extraordinary organisms that concern this part of the story.

Phages are beautiful to observe; they are also ubiquitous. Essentially, where there are bacteria, there are phages. They are in our guts, on our skin, in our mouth, and in our nose and throat. They are in soil and seawater. They are relatively simple in structure, and they resemble nothing so much as prototype computer game space invader monsters from the 1970s. They are simply genetic material – nucleic acid – surrounded by a protein coat. The process of a phage attacking a bacterium has been observed and filmed in real time on many occasions, and the images are engrossing. The protein frame of a bacteriophage looks as if it is made from Meccano, the engineering kit for children. It has an almost cylindrical body supported on articulated, jointed legs. An attacking phage lands on its victim – for which it is specific – like the early Apollo landing craft. It then gently probes the surface of the cell for the correct receptor. At this moment, it triggers the reaction that the phage is searching for. Its legs contract and a needle-like protuberance squirts the phage's contents into the bacterium.

Exactly like viruses that affect us, once the phages have injected their genetic material into their bacteria, then they very often take over the synthetic machinery of their victims. They force the bacteria to make more phage particles, even ordering them to produce enzymes that will cause their hosts to dissolve themselves from the inside out. Thus, the bacteria can release the freshly made bacterial viruses, bursting in the process.

The fact that each phage generally has only one type of victim has been very important in the past for scientists, and may yet become so again. Suppose you are investigating an outbreak of a disease caused by bacteria. Bacteria are in some respects like breeds of dog. They may belong to the same species but be sub-grouped into breeds; in the case of bacteria, strains. You want to know if all the victims of your outbreak are affected by the same strain of your bacterial species, because you want to try to identify and control the source. You have specimens growing on your laboratory agar plates, but they all appear identical. How can you distinguish among them? Nowadays, we can type them by genetic methods, but in the past we did not have such technology available. We did know about phages, though. It is a simple matter to culture your bacteria upon a plate and then drip a small quantity of phage onto them; most phages will only kill their own target. You can then identify your strain by noting which phage kills which bug. For many years this was the most reliable means of identifying strains of bacteria; MRSA, for example, would have had an associated phage number until very recently.

Once you know the phage type of the bacterium you are dealing with, there is nothing to stop you using it to treat your patient. If the infection is on a superficial part of the body, then nothing could be simpler. The solution of phage can just be sprayed on. The beauty of phage therapy is that it cannot easily outlive its victim. Once all of its targets are dead, then it cannot reproduce. It may survive in the right conditions, but it cannot reproduce and thus poses no risk. It cannot damage cells in the human body, because we lack the necessary receptors to which it may attach and in which it may squirt its genetic contents. Phages that spill over into the bloodstream are simply picked up and eradicated like any other alien material. This advantage is two-edged; it means that deeper-seated infections cannot easily be treated by phage, because the body's natural defences will annihilate them before they can reproduce. If you can get a needle into the site of infection, you may have a chance. Intravenous therapy, of the sort that is used for antibiotics, will generally be doomed to failure. The phage's specific need to infect its particular strain of victim is also limiting. Not every infection is caused by a single strain of bacterium, and eradicating one strain may permit other phage-resistant strains to emerge, exactly as happens with antibiotics. That is not to say that they have no other uses; experiments have been carried out with eradication of cholera in water supplies through phage. However, the advent of effective antibiotics really terminated interest in phages as treatment in the 1940s. Twenty-five years earlier, however, things were very different.

Phages were discovered almost simultaneously by two scientists working on opposite sides of the Atlantic: Frederick Twort in England in 1915, and the extraordinary and complex aristocrat Félix d'Herelle in Canada in 1917. D'Herelle identified phage in, of all places, locust diarrhoea. He was a passionate communist, and he presented his discoveries as a gift to his hero Stalin. He was thus invited to join the Eliava Institute in Tbilisi, Georgia in 1934. Its scientists subsequently supplied the Red Army with phage active against dysentery during the Second World War. The Institute is credited with a contribution to the Soviet war effort comparable to that of Fleming with penicillin. D'Herelle was the subsequent hero of a book about his life by Sinclair Lewis called *Arrowsmith*; in this fictional version of events, phage therapy failed to gain acceptance because the hero, in trying to cure plague in the West Indies, failed to use proper scientific technique.

Lewis's novel has a prophetic echo in the world's subsequent indifference to phage therapy. We have mentioned in passing how few innovations have arisen in agents active against the Quiet Killers in the states of the former Soviet Union. There is more to this than simply absence of the profit incentive. Apart from the unfortunate fact that most scientific research published in any language other than English tends to be ignored in the West, Soviet scientific advances have been disastrously contaminated by the ideologically driven dogma of one man. That man's name was Trofim Lysenko. Since Lysenko, no Soviet science has ever been taken very seriously. With a supreme irony that will become more apparent as the story progresses, the nature of this dogma was the wistful and forlorn faith of many communists in an obscure and discredited pseudo-scientific creed called Lamarckism. I propose to examine this tangential aspect of the phage story in a little detail; it is this as much as anything that has denied the West the real benefits of the Eliava Institute for sixty years. Furthermore, there has been a further excruciating twist to the story from modern times. Without understanding this part of the story, much of the richness of that irony would be lost.

Communists like Stalin would have loved Lamarckism to be true. In fact, Stalin would have loved it to be true so much that Soviet scientists who espoused Darwinism were sent to the gulags. Put simply, it is the belief that non-hereditary traits may be passed on to the next generation. For example, giraffes find themselves in a changing environment in which they can only survive by eating leaves high up on trees. So they stretch their necks to reach the leaves, and this stretching and the desire to stretch are passed on to later generations. As a result, a species of animal which originally had short necks evolved into a species with long necks. This is a direct contrast to Darwinian evolution. The communists loved the idea because it would mean that all men truly might become equal; with adequate education, qualities such as intelligence would become hereditary, human attainments would level, and social justice ensue. Exactly as some right-wing ideologues grasp at Darwin to justify ruthless and exclusionist social policies, so socialists would ruefully point at Lamarckism.

The problem with Lamarckism is that it is quite simply wrong. This is not a question of opinion, in a Creationist versus Darwinist sense, but of applied fact. The most reliable test of any scientific hypothesis is whether its principles are supported by experiment. Under Lysenko's guidance, the results were predictable: the steady deterioration of Soviet biology, and the failure of mass agricultural experiments based on his ideology. Lysenko was not denounced by the Soviet scientific community until 1965, more than ten years after Stalin had died; by then, it was of course far too late for the reputation of Soviet science. That reputation was not helped by the next peculiar twist to this part of the story, the fate of George Eliava, the founder of the Georgian phage institute. Eliava was something of a playboy. He dallied with a woman who was the favourite of Lavrenty Beria, head of Stalin's secret police, and was shot in 1937 on a trumped-up pretext. D'Herelle's fantastic discoveries were thus ignored in the west for decades.

In a peculiar post-collapse of communism twist of fate, in 1996, a Canadian venture capitalist named Caisey Harlingten spotted an article about the work of the Eliava Institute at Tbilisi, Georgia in an in-flight magazine. Aware that we might need to revisit apparently redundant treatment strategies, Harlingten realised that his fellow Canadian had been onto something remarkable. He tried to establish cooperation between American venture capitalists and the Georgians. Sadly, there was something of a culture clash. The Eliava Institute was crumbling, its ancient laboratories in desperate need of rebuilding after the collapse of communism. That is not to say that the Institute had been perfectly run under the communists; D'Herelle's own quarters had been commandeered by the KGB as their local HQ. Most of the Institute's enormous and almost irreplaceable library of phage had been lost due to power cuts and equipment failure. Understandably, the scientists and directors were woefully naïve in the ruthless ways of capitalism. The East–West cooperative Institute set up at Tbilisi folded almost immediately. There is now a thriving institute of research into phage in Seattle, while the Eliava continues to crumble. Its directors feel that their research and experience were quite simply stolen.

Practical applications for phage are now rapidly developing. A kind of super-bandage impregnated with seven phages that can kill all the likely bacteria to infect wounds has emerged; it is called PhageBioderm. It is being developed by an American company called Intralytix. Such usage is already under investigation for eradication of resistant hospital bacteria. Modern technology may be capable of modifying these fascinating beasts into something even more useful. In fact, although it was stated earlier that phages, when injected intravenously, are destroyed by the body's immune system, some phages can mutate; and when they do so, it can be into a form that can survive inside the body. They may then be injected through other routes; for example, into the abdomen. A mutation within the phage's own genes is required for this to take place. Such a mutation has been invoked artificially by repeatedly passing phages through the body and harvesting those that survive. The nature of this mutation may be quite straightforward and easy to reproduce; it may then be possible to engineer genetically phages that are capable of killing bacteria when injected intravenously. The Eliava Institute claims to have just such a phage which is active against MRSA. For this to work, we would still need to know for certain precisely which strain of bacterium was causing the infection, to a degree which was never usually necessary with bacteria. Phages may also be useful for decontaminating inanimate surfaces which harbour dangerous bacteria.

The ability of phages to mutate is also the source of one of the potential hazards of their use. We have mentioned their inherent capacity for mutation. Like most viruses, they are prone to it. A mutant phage might conceivably do harm to a person, but such an event has not as yet been recorded. However, phages have another means of altering their genes which may be more worrying. Remember, they work by hijacking the machinery of a target cell and then using that machinery to reproduce themselves. At certain stages in their life cycle, there will be naked phage genetic material under construction adjacent to the genes of the target bacterium. Suppose our phage infects a bacterium which has the genes for multiple bacterial resistance, or production of a deadly toxin, or some other property we would sooner avoid. It is entirely plausible that the phage might pick up that gene while under construction and transfer it into the next bacterium it infects. That bacterium might also have developed phage resistance. The phage then transfers its genetic load including our danger gene into a bacterium that survives. This may seem far-fetched, but remember that each bacterium may produce many thousands of phages as it dies, and each colony of bacteria may contain billions of individual organisms. The odds are really in favour of this sort of event, and indeed phages have been shown to transfer genes between bacteria.

The fact that it is restricted in its targets; its capacity for mutation; its capacity for transferring potentially dangerous genes, all limit the potential usefulness of the phage. Nonetheless, like an army that has run out of bullets, we may have to use technology like the phage as a sort of hand-to-hand combat, a bayonet charge if you will. It may be possible to exploit phages a little further yet, by extracting protein products from them that are toxic to bacteria. This has been the approach at the Montreal-based PhageTech in a collaboration with McGill University. All of this means two cheers for the bacteriophage.

* * *

We should look to our tears next, because fortunately for us they provide other avenues to explore in our all-out war against the Quiet Killers. These are the so-called anti-microbial peptides. They are also known as natural defence peptides; as defensins; and by a number of other titles, including cathelicidins. When the same substances have so many names, you can be sure that they are the subject of excited research by multiple groups of scientists. They can be found in many of our body fluids – sweat, saliva, semen and tears – and most body surfaces, including the gut, lung and genital tract. The skin of our mouths and tongues, and right through to our anuses, is covered by these simple but useful proteins. Like many other aspects of our immune systems, they are intimately involved with allergies. For example, absence of one, called LL37, is involved with allergic dermatitis and resulting skin infections.

These chemicals, which can appear in many guises and with many different structures, can be synthesised artificially in the lab and used as treatments. They have many advantages. First, they have evolved as a first-line defence against infection. As such, much of the 'thinking' involved with their design has been done for us. Second, because they are natural products of our own cells they are less likely to do us harm. This rule is not absolute; our bodies produce many substances which are potentially toxic if they are in the wrong place. Many of these are produced in response to infections. Nevertheless, defensins look promising. If I had to select one new technology that was likely to be 'product rich', it would be this one.

Hope for the future from traditional drug development would seem, therefore, to be at best qualified. There is better news, though. New technologies have meant that we no longer have to rely on the empirical, almost serendipitous approach to new drugs bequeathed to us by Fleming. For many years, the best way to look for a new antibiotic was to drop a flask into a sewage outfall and screen all the bugs you found there to see if they produced anything useful. They would then be tested to see if they were safe for animals, and then humans. With luck, and by testing enough compounds, you might find such a new drug; however, many hundreds had to be tested and rejected for just one success.

Science, though, has moved on. We can now approach the problem from the other end. We understand ever-increasing amounts about the life cycles, metabolic processes and even the genetic structure of many of the Quiet Killers. This allows us to identify processes that are peculiar to them, and thereby to design substances that are toxic to them but not to us. Whole new classes of antibiotics have been developed using this approach. Scientists even congratulated themselves that they had been so cunning that the Quiet Killers would never be able to develop resistance to these entirely new compounds. Artificial 'designer' compounds would be far harder for microbes to outwit. Such a class of artificially designed drugs is the oxazolidinones, the best known of which is Linezolid.

Linezolid was carefully designed as a molecule that would stop bacteria producing proteins. Although it is relatively limited in its activity, it has proven extremely useful in treating MRSA and similar infections. As it is not a naturally occurring substance, it was confidently expected that resistance could never emerge. Sadly – and predictably – this has not been the case. Linezolid resistance has appeared in several places in the world.

If you're desperate and you can't think of a new idea, then why not just tinker with an old one? From the very first days of antibiotics, minor adjustments to the structure of drug molecules has been hugely fruitful. Fleming's original penicillin was not really practically useful until its structure had been modified slightly. Whole groups of antibiotics have now been developed that simply amend a basic structure, adding a molecule here and trimming one there. It would, of course, be tedious for the purposes of this chapter to go into the precise detail of this chemical tailoring; the patterns of the molecules seem identical to the untutored eye. What is striking when examining pictures of them is how amazing it is that one simple atom of fluorine, say, when tacked on to an otherwise identical and bog-standard antibiotic, can totally transform its activity or toxicity. How on earth do they do it?

The ingenuity and imagination that scientists use can only give us hope for the future. For example, Professor Andrew Myers of Harvard uses large-scale fermentation to try to synthesise new antibiotics from a basic product. The antibiotic he is interested in is tetracycline, itself a fermentation product of a microbe. Fermentation has always been used in its synthesis; the brilliantly different approach Myers has taken is to start the process with a synthetic molecule. He has generated entirely new potential antibiotics as a consequence.

Some drugs which were once virtually discarded have found a new lease of life from this sort of fine-tuning. Thalidomide is an excellent example. Some readers may not be familiar with the thalidomide story. It is worth recapping briefly. This was a drug widely prescribed in pregnancy for morning sickness during the 1960s and '70s. Tragically, however, it had a catastrophic propensity for causing birth defects, particularly stunted limb growth. The drug was nearly abandoned; this was a shame because thalidomide has some uses when ranged against some of the most deadly infections, including leprosy and TB. What may have salvaged the drug is a phenomenon called chirality. Images of drug molecules are hard enough to decipher and distinguish. Chirality makes things even worse. Basically, molecules may sometimes take one of two forms – left- or right-handed. More often than not this doesn't matter, and most drug production makes no effort to separate the two. The resulting mixture of left- and right-handed forms is known as racemic. Sometimes, though, the right-handed molecule may behave so differently from the left-handed type that you may want only one or the other. So it has been with thalidomide; the laevo-isomer (left-handed molecule) is dangerous, while the dextro-isomer (right-handed molecule) is blameless. It wasn't until the logistics of producing one or the other exclusively were worked out that it became possible to produce 'safe' thalidomide for the treatment of diseases such as TB and leprosy. This refinement earned its discoverers the 2001 Nobel Prize.

Deciphering the genetic structure of the Quiet Killers has been less fruitful in developing new drugs. The approach is 'target-rich, product-poor', in the buzz phrase. We will discuss why in a moment, and it will become clear that now scientists have understood those reasons they have been able to move on to be more productive. However, it is worth explaining how some antiviral drugs work at this juncture so that this point may be clearly understood. The genetic code of all known organisms (apart from prions) is made up of DNA and RNA. Both are composed of extended chains of building blocks called bases. While new DNA or RNA is being constructed, each base has to have the right 'hook' on it to allow the next base to attach. Some antiviral agents work by mimicking the structure of building blocks of DNA, but with the important difference that the 'hook' is missing. These are the so-called 'chain terminators'. Aciclovir, the drug for cold sores and genital herpes, is the first and commonest antiviral of this type. Many drugs active against HIV work on the same principle. The reason they terminate viral DNA and RNA chains is that viruses are sloppier in identifying and using bases than more complex organisms; our cells are too picky to accept the base mimic.

You might have thought that knowing the key to life, the genetic code, of an organism would allow us to target it highly effectively and specifically. The simple fact is that this has not been true, so far at any rate. The example given above, chain termination, works because of the sloppiness of the virus in examining and incorporating bases into its growing DNA or RNA chain. It does not rely on knowing the genetic code of the virus. Trying to attack the Quiet Killers by reading their gene sequence is a bit like planning a bombing raid on a city by reading its telephone directory. It was all far more complex than it seemed at first. The traditional view of genetics was that a sequence of bases formed a code, and that the code was predictable. The genes of this code could be transcribed into a product, which was a protein. The convention was that each code sequence represented a single protein. However, when scientists began to look in detail at the proteins that were present in even simple bacteria, they found an amazing thing – *there were more proteins than genes*. The action of genes is far more complex than originally thought – two genes can act together to produce a number of different possible products, for instance. The gene may work more economically by starting the code-reading process at different points along the chain. Proteins may be modified by other proteins after they have been synthesised. Some genes may not be translated into proteins at all, or only under particular conditions – for example, toxic proteins may only be produced when the bug is actually causing disease.

Creative, artful humankind has moved on, however. We are no longer restricted to simply examining the pure sequence of DNA or RNA and best-guessing what the products might be. Now we can break up our target germ and examine in detail every single protein product. The means of doing this has become so advanced that it may be performed on a tiny chip called a microarray. Thousands of proteins may be compared almost instantaneously by computer. This technology, broadly known as proteomics, has revolutionised many aspects of research into the Quiet Killers. Its most basic application is in the art of identification. Suppose you want to know whether the strain of MRSA that is creating havoc in your hospital is the same as the one which is troubling St Elsewhere's up the road. Where once you might have tried the effective but comparatively slow and imprecise phage-typing, now you can drip your bug onto a microarray and have an answer within hours. You could also sequence the gene, but it seems that proteomics is quicker, easier and cheaper.

The potential benefits are far more exciting. An excellent way of killing a bug is to target some aspect that is unique to it. Most antibiotics work in this way; sulphonamides, for example, work by interfering with the requirement of bacteria to generate their own folic acid. Humans can absorb this vitamin from their diet, and so are immune to drugs which disrupt that particular pathway. Proteomics gives us just the right clues to such potential weaknesses in the Quiet Killers. We can deduce specific pathways and products, and then we can target them. Many conventionally designed antibiotics act by disrupting the synthesis of proteins; proteomics offers us the possibility of attacking these more selectively. One advantage of this might be reduced toxicity. An antibiotic that will only affect particular microbial pathways is probably less likely to damage human cells. I say 'probably' because the Linezolid experience has been minatory in this respect. This antibiotic, widely believed to be safe, has now been shown to cause nerve damage and even blindness. A second advantage might be in preventing a bacterium from producing its toxic product. This would be in preference to killing it, as we would simply turn our Quiet Killer into a Silent Pacifist. If the toxic products that prevent them being digested by our white blood cells are switched off, then they will once again be vulnerable to that natural process. Designing drugs like this is in fact like choosing exact addresses from the telephone directory in the city that you wish to bomb, thus leaving the innocent intact.

On the down side, we have yet to hear of a truly successful antibiotic that has been successfully derived from any of these new technologies. While it may be true that the last great hope for a magic bullet – gene analysis – has led to little in the way of new anti-infectives, that doesn't mean it isn't vital in the battle against the Quiet Killers. Monitoring patterns of resistance to HIV drugs relies very heavily on analysis of mutations in the gene. My prediction is that proteomics will do at least as much. Proteomics offers us real new insights into the behaviour of our ancient enemies, and it is hard to see how that cannot bear fruit. Questions such as whether this bacterium is producing the protein that causes resistance to my antibiotics can be answered more swiftly and simply than ever before. Here's another example. Fungal infections are a major cause of illness and death among people with cancers and leukaemias whose protective white cells have been deliberately annihilated by chemotherapy. One of the most challenging diagnostic dilemmas in medicine is deciding whether the very common fungus you have found on your patient is an innocent pacifist or a Quiet Killer. Probably half of the very expensive and toxic anti-fungal drugs that are prescribed are given to people who do not have a serious fungal infection. Proteomics can tell us whether the invader is armed and dangerous or not, because certain proteins will only be produced in disease. Furthermore, proteomics can be reversed to look at the host. Our cells will only switch on certain proteins in the presence of illness. We will soon be able to answer questions such as, does our patient with a mysterious illness for which no cause can be found have an infection or not?, without actually having to find the concealed Quiet Killer. We will know it by its proteomic reflection.

So we end on a note of qualified optimism. Proteomics, gene analysis, bacteriophages, defensins and the rest will certainly be at the cutting edge of research and seem certain to offer us useful weapons. Whether they will deliver the haymaker killer blows that we took for granted in the twentieth century is another matter; it would be rash to predict. What is almost certain, though, is that such research will benefit the citizens of the developed world far more than our less fortunate cousins in the poorer countries. The real tragedy of the Quiet Killers is that we already have the technology to make effective inroads into infectious diseases in those countries. It has been argued that Waterloo would have been an easier victory for Wellington and Blücher had they used longbows against Napoleon instead of muskets. Longbows are cheaper, quicker to reload, easier to build and repair, and more accurate. It is exactly so in our war against disease in poorer countries. New technology is not always better technology. A combination of poverty, political instability, war, famine and simple failure of collective will have paralysed our onslaught. Yet such simple technology as proper mosquito nets could save many thousands from malaria; clean drinking water could save millions. That isn't to say we shouldn't be ardently pursuing novel and exciting means of assault on our targets. I have observed the deaths of patients infected with diseases that were once treatable. There really is little to choose in those circumstances between us with our MRI scanners, intensive care units, and ultra-modern operating theatres, and the barefoot doctor or even the shaman.

Sources and Further Reading

Rather than providing detailed, numbered references which might interrupt the text, I have listed below books that readers may find interesting, as well as some of my sources. I have tried not to include too many references to primary research journals, as they are often not accessible to the general reader; I have done so where there is no alternative, widely available source. Much of the information in the text is gleaned from years of experience in infectious diseases and microbiology, rather than detailed searching of textbooks and primary sources. Use was also made of a series of lectures at the University of London between 2003 and 2005 as part of a Master's Degree.

For overall technical reference, the following books were invaluable, but are detailed and lengthy textbooks.

Cook, G. and Zumla, A., *Manson's Tropical Diseases*, London, W.B. Saunders, 2002

Hoeprich, P.D., *Infectious Diseases: A Guide to the Understanding and Management of Infectious Processes*, Philadelphia, 1st edn, Harper & Row, 1972

Mandell, G.L., Bennett, J.E. and Dolin, R., *Mandell Douglas and Bennett's Principles and Practice of Infectious Diseases*, New York, Churchill Livingstone, 1995

Introduction

Dormandy, T., *The White Death: A History of Tuberculosis*, New York, New York University Press, 2000

Fraser, A., *Cromwell, Our Chief of Men*, London, Phoenix Press, 2002

Nissel, M., *People Count: A History of the General Register Office*, London, HMSO, 1987

Quorum sensing: for a readable and informative account, visit the website http://www.nottingham.ac.uk/quorum/

Chapter One

Brock, T.D., *Robert Koch: A Life in Medicine and Bacteriology*, Washington, American Society of Microbiology, 2000

Halliday, S., *The Great Stink of London: Sir Joseph Bazalgette and the Cleansing of the Victorian Metropolis*, Stroud, Sutton, 2001

Pasteur, L. and Lister, J., *Germ Theory and Its Applications to Medicine & On the Antiseptic Principle of the Practice of Surgery*, New York, reprint, Prometheus Books, 1996

Ryan, F., *Tuberculosis: The Greatest Story Never Told*, London, Swift, 1992

Sass, E.J., Gottfried, G. and Sorem, A., *Polio's Legacy: An Oral History*, Lanham, Maryland, University Press of America, 1996

Snow, J., *Snow on cholera; being a reprint of two papers*, New York, Hafner Pub. Co., January 1965

Yount, L., *Antoni Van Leeuwenhoek: First to See Microscopic Life* (Great Minds of Science), Berkeley Heights, NJ, Enslow Publishers, 2001

Chapter Two

Alcorn, K., 'EU Consensus Lacking on Needle Exchange', *Journal of the International Association of Physicians in AIDS Care*, 4:6 (1998), 37

Bellaby, P., 'Has the UK Government Lost the Battle over MMR?', *British Medical Journal* 330 (2005), 552–3

Cook, G.C., *From the Greenwich Hulks to Old St Pancras. A History of Tropical Disease in London*, London, Athlone Press, 1992

Despommier, D. and Demarest, R.J., *West Nile Story*, New York, Apple Trees Productions, 2001

Reiter, P., 'From Shakespeare to Defoe: Malaria in England in the Little Ice Age', *Emerging Infectious Diseases*, 6:1 (2000), 1–11

Simms, I. *et al.*, 'The Re-emergence of Syphilis in the United Kingdom: The New Epidemic Phases', *Sexually Transmitted Diseases*, 32:4 (2005), 220–6

Statistics on worldwide incidence of sexually transmitted diseases, visit the website http://www.avert.org/stdstatisticsworldwide.htm

Voltaire, *Candide*, trans. J. Butt, London, rev. edn, Penguin, 1950

Chapter Three

Bloom, B. and Lambert, P.H., *The Vaccine Book*, New York, Academic Press, 2000

Cook, G.C., 'Influence of Diarrhoeal Disease on Military and Naval Campaigns', *Journal of the Royal Society of Medicine*, 94:2 (2001), 95–7

Frieden, T.R., Fujiwara, P.I., Washko, R.M. and Hamburg, M.A., 'Tuberculosis in New York City: Turning the Tide', *New England Journal of Medicine*, 333 (1995), 229–33

Rocco, F., *Quinine: Malaria and the Quest for a Cure that Changed the World*, London, reprint edn, Harper Perennial, 2004

Smith, F.B., *The Retreat of Tuberculosis, 1850–1950*, London, Croom Helm, 1988

For information on new HIV vaccines, see
www.niaid.nih.gov/daids/vaccine/concepts.htm

Chapter Four

Cartwright, F. and Biddiss, M., *Disease and History*, Stroud, Sutton, 2004

Crosby, A.W., *Ecological Imperialism: The Biological Expansion of Europe, 900–1900*, Cambridge, Cambridge University Press, 1986

McNeill, W., *Plagues and Peoples*, New York, rev. edn, Anchor, 1977

Pierce, J.R. and Writer J.V., *Yellow Jack: How Yellow Fever Ravaged America and Walter Reed Discovered its Deadly Secrets*, Hoboken, NJ, Wiley, 2005

Woodham-Smith, C., *The Great Hunger: Ireland 1845–1849*, Harmondsworth, Penguin, 1979

Chapter Five

Alibek, K. and Handelman, S., *Biohazard: The Chilling True Story of the Largest Covert Biological Weapons Program in the World – Told from Inside by the Man Who Ran It*, New York, Delta, 2000

Barnaby, W., *The Plague Makers. The Secret World of Biological Warfare*, London, Vision, 1997

Derbes, V.J., 'De Mussis and the Great Plague of 1348. A Forgotten Episode of Bacteriological Warfare', *Journal of the American Medical Association*, 196 (1966), 59–62

Gruzinski, S., *The Conquest of Mexico*, Cambridge, Polity, 1993

Hopkins, D.R., *Princes and Peasants: Smallpox in History*, Chicago, Chicago University Press, 1983

Knight, B., 'Ricin: A Potent Homicidal Poison', *British Medical Journal*, 1 (1979), 350–1

Meselson, M. *et al.*, 'The Sverdlovsk Anthrax Outbreak of 1979', *Science*, 266:5188 (18 November 1994), 1202–8

Snowden, F., *The Conquest of Malaria: Italy, 1900–1962*, Yale, Yale University Press, 2006

Torok, T.J. *et al.*, 'A Large Community Outbreak of Salmonellosis Caused by Intentional Contamination of Restaurant Salad bars', *Journal of the American Medical Association*, 278 (1997), 389–95

UN, 'UNSCOM and the UNSCOM experience in Iraq', *Politics and the Life Sciences*, 14:2 (August 1995), 230–5

WHO, *The Global Eradication of Smallpox*, Geneva, World Health Organization, 1980

Chapter Six

Adlercreutz, H. *et al.*, 'Studies on the Role of Intestinal Bacteria in Metabolism of Synthetic and Natural Steroid Hormones', *Journal of Steroid Biochemistry*, 20:1 (1984), 217–29

Alm, J.S. *et al.*, 'Atopy in Children of Families with Anthroposophic Lifestyle', *The Lancet*, 353 (1 May 1999), 1485

Bjorksten, B. *et al.*, 'Prevalence of Childhood Asthma, Rhinitis and Eczema in Scandinavia and Eastern Europe', *European Respiratory Journal* 12:2 (1998), 432–7

Farooqi, I.S. and Hopkin, J.M., 'Early Childhood Infection and Atopic Disorder', *Thorax*, 53 (1998), 927

Margulis, L., *Symbiotic Planet: A New Look at Evolution*, New York, Basic Books, 2000

Marra, F. *et al.*, 'Does Antibiotic Exposure during Infancy Lead to Development of Asthma? A Systematic Review and Metaanalysis', *Chest*, 129:3 (2006), 610–18

Matricardi, P.M. *et al.*, 'Exposure to Foodborne and Orofecal Microbes versus Airborne Viruses in relation to Atopy and Allergic Asthma: Epidemiological Study', *British Medical Journal*, 320:7232 (2000), 412–17

——, 'Cross Sectional Retrospective Study of Prevalence of Atopy among Italian Military Students with Antibodies Against Hepatitis A Virus', *British Medical Journal*, 314:7086 (1997), 999–1003

Stanford, J.L. *et al.*, 'How Environmental Mycobacteria may Predetermine the Protective Efficacy of BCG', *Tubercle*, 62:1 (1981), 55–62

Stapleton, J.T., Xiang, J. and Williams, C.F., 'HIV and GB Virus C Coinfection', *The Lancet Infectious Diseases*, 6:4 (2006), 187–8

Summers, R.W. *et al.*, 'Trichuris Suis Therapy for Active Ulcerative Colitis: A Randomized Controlled Trial', *Gastroenterology*, 128:4 (2005), 825–32

Chapter Seven

Barry, J.M., *The Great Influenza: The Epic Story of the Deadliest Plague In History*, New York, Viking Adult, 2004

Bell, W.G., *The Great Plague in London in 1665*, London, John Lane, 1924

Crichton, M., *The Andromeda Strain*, New York, Knopf, 1969

Crosby, A.W., *Epidemic and Peace 1918*, London, Greenwood, 1976

Drancourt, M. *et al.*, 'Detection of 400-year-old *Yersinia pestis* DNA in Human Dental Pulp: An Approach to the Diagnosis of Ancient Septicaemia', *Proceedings of the National Academy of Science of the USA*, 95:21 (1998), 12637–40

Fenner, F. and Fantini, B., *Biological Control of Vertebrate Pests: The History of Myxomatosis – An Experiment in Evolution*, Geneva, CABI, 1999

Hayes, R.A. and Richardson, B.J., 'Biological Control of the Rabbit in Australia: Lessons Not Learned?', *Trends in Microbiology*, 9:9 (2001), 459–60

Hirst, L.F., *The Conquest of Plague*, Oxford, Clarendon Press, 1953

Huang, Y. *et al.*, 'The Role of a Mutant CCR5 Allele in HIV-1 Transmission and Disease Progression', *Nature Medicine* 2:11 (1996), 1240–3

Prentice, M.B., Gilbert, T. and Cooper A., 'Was the Black Death Caused by *Yersinia pestis*?', *The Lancet Infectious Diseases*, 4:2 (2004), 72

Rigg, J.M. (trans.), *The Decameron Of Giovanni Boccaccio*, London, privately published, 1921

Chapter Eight

Dawkins, R., *The Blind Watchmaker: Why the Evidence of Evolution Reveals a Universe Without Design*, Eastbourne, Gardners Books, 1990

Eldridge, B.F. and Edman, J.D. (eds), *Medical Entomology: A Textbook on Public Health and Veterinary Problems Caused by Arthropods*, 2nd edn, New York, Springer, 2003

Ewald, P.W., *Plague Time: How Stealth Infections Cause Cancer, Heart Disease, and Other Deadly Ailments*, New York, Free Press, 2000

Jeffs, B., 'A Clinical Guide to Viral Haemorrhagic Fevers: Ebola, Marburg and Lassa', *Tropical Doctor*, 36:1 (2006), 1–4

Service, M., *Medical Entomology for Students*, 3rd edn, Cambridge, Cambridge University Press, 2004

Chapter Nine

Abraham, T., *Twenty-First Century Plague: The Story of SARS*, Baltimore, Maryland, Johns Hopkins University Press, 2005

Das, P., 'Antibiotic Resistance in Europe', *The Lancet Infectious Diseases*, 3:7 (2003), 398

Hilton, D.A., 'Pathogenesis and Prevalence of Variant Creutzfeldt-Jakob Disease', *Journal of Pathology*, 208:2 (2006), 134–41

Parker, J.N. and Parker, P.M. (eds), *The Official Patient's Sourcebook on Tropical Spastic Paraparesis*, San Diego, Icon Health Publications, 2002

Singer, R.S. *et al.*, 'Antibiotic Resistance – The Interplay between Antibiotic Use in Animals and Human Beings', *The Lancet Infectious Diseases*, 3:1 (2003), 47–51

Todd, N.V. *et al.*, 'Cerebroventricular Infusion of Pentosan Polysulphate in Human Variant Creutzfeldt-Jakob Disease', *Journal of Infection*, 50:5 (2005), 394–6

Van Zwanenberg, P. and Millstone, E., *BSE: Risk, Science, and Governance*, Oxford, Oxford University Press, 2005

For the CJD surveillance unit in Edinburgh, visit http://www.cjd.ed.ac.uk/

Chapter Ten

Anon., *CDC Outbreak of Hendra-like virus – Malaysia and Singapore, 1998–1999*, MMWR 48 (1999), 265–9

Askari, F.K., *Hepatitis C: The Silent Epidemic*, London, HarperCollins, 2001

Chua, K.B. *et al.*, 'Fatal Encephalitis due to Nipah Virus among Pig-farmers in Malaysia', *The Lancet*, 354 (1999), 1257–9

Fraser, D.W. *et al.*, 'Legionnaires' Disease: Description of an Epidemic of Pneumonia', *New England Journal of Medicine*, 297:22 (1977), 1189–97

Garrett, L., *The Coming Plague: Newly Emerging Diseases in a World Out of Balance*, New York, Farrar Straus Giroux, 1994

Grmek, M.D., *History of AIDS*, trans. R.C. Maulitz and J. Duffin, Princeton, Princeton University Press, 1993

Hooper, E. and Hamilton, W., *The River: A Journey to the Source of HIV and AIDS*, Boston, Little, Brown, 1999

Wolfe, N.D., 'Naturally Acquired Simian Retrovirus Infections in Central African Hunters', *The Lancet*, 363:9413 (2004), 932–7

Chapter Eleven

Calendar, R.L., *The Bacteriophages*, Oxford, Oxford University Press, 2006

Campbell, W.C., *Ivermectin and Abamectin*, New York, Springer, 1989

Hancock, R.E., 'Cationic Peptides: Effectors in Innate Immunity and Novel Antimicrobials', *The Lancet Infectious Diseases*, 1:3 (2001), 156–64

——, 'Mechanisms of Action of Newer Antibiotics for Gram-positive Pathogens', *The Lancet Infectious Diseases*, 5:4 (2005), 209–18

Salyers, A.A. and Whitt, D.D., *Revenge of the Microbes: How Bacterial Resistance is Undermining the Antibiotic Miracle*, Washington, ASM Press, 2005

Twyman, R.M., *Principles of Proteomics*, Abingdon, Oxon, Advanced Text Series, BIOS Scientific Publishers, 2004

Index

Index